Healthy Eating Is the First Step in Taking Care of Your Diabetes

If you have diabetes, you do not need to eat special foods. The foods that are good for everyone are also good for you. This booklet can help you choose healthy foods in appropriate portion sizes to keep your blood glucose (blood sugar) levels within your target range.

A healthy Eating Plan:
- Includes foods such as vegetables, fruits, whole grains, legumes (beans, lentils, and peas), low-fat or fat-free milk and milk products, seafood, lean meats and poultry, and nuts and seeds.
- Limits foods that are high in sodium (salt), solid fats, and added sugars.
- Does not include *trans* fats.
- Helps you control your blood glucose levels and meet your weight goals.

Healthy Eating and Your Blood Glucose Levels

To keep your blood glucose within your target range, it is important to monitor your blood glucose levels and balance three things:
- The amounts and types of foods you eat (especially carbohydrate foods)
- Your physical activity
- The insulin your body makes or the insulin you inject

When you keep your blood glucose levels within your target range, you will feel better and lower your risk of diabetes complications.

The energy your body needs is measured in calories. Calories come from three nutrients found in the foods you eat:
- Carbohydrate
- Protein
- Fat

Your body needs insulin to use these nutrients correctly. Insulin is made by the pancreas. When you eat foods, especially those that contain carbohydrate, they turn into glucose (a type of sugar). Glucose is the energy source for the cells in your body. Insulin helps get the glucose into the cells. When a person has diabetes, the pancreas does not make insulin or does not make enough insulin to get glucose into the body's cells. If you have a condition called insulin resistance, your pancreas makes insulin but your body does not use it very well. When you have diabetes or insulin resistance, your blood glucose levels may rise too high.

To keep your blood glucose levels within your target range, it is helpful to eat about the same amount of food, especially carbohydrate, at about the same times each day. However, if you take multiple daily injections of insulin or use an insulin pump to control your blood glucose levels, you have more freedom to vary the amounts you eat and your mealtimes. Regardless of how you manage your diabetes, plan to spread your meals and snacks throughout the day. Your registered dietitian nutritionist (RDN) can help you decide the timing and sizes of meals and snacks that are right for you.

Take care to not skip any meals. Skipping meals may make it harder for you to control your appetite and weight. If you use insulin or certain glucose-lowering medications, skipping meals may also lead to low blood glucose levels.

Healthy Eating, Physical Activity, and Your Weight

You get energy (calories) from the food you eat. Your body uses energy when you breathe, sit, walk, or move (physical activity). Your weight stays the same when the energy in (calories from the food you eat) equals the energy out (the energy your body uses). You gain weight when you take in more energy (calories) than your body uses. This extra energy is stored as weight (fat). When you take in fewer calories from food than your body uses as energy, you lose weight because your body burns off stored energy. Therefore, you can lose weight by eating less and/or by increasing physical activity. If you are at a healthy weight, you can maintain that weight by balancing the energy you take in from food and the energy you use for physical activity. Your RDN can help you set your calorie and physical activity goals.

Planning Healthy Meals

The Eating Plan on the inside of the back cover of this booklet can help you plan healthy meals. You and your RDN will fill in the Eating Plan together. Use the Eating Plan to help you select the number of choices from each food list in this booklet that is right for you at each meal and snack. In your plan, the number of choices from each food list is based on your calorie and nutrient needs, your lifestyle and usual schedule of eating, and your diabetes management plan.

The food lists in this booklet group together foods that have about the same amount of carbohydrate, protein, fat, and calories. The term choice is used to describe a certain quantity of food within a group of similar foods.

- Foods on the **Starch** list, **Fruits** list, and **Milk and Milk Substitutes** list are similar because they contain 12 to 15 grams of carbohydrate per choice.
- Foods on the Starchy Vegetable list (part of the **Starch** list and including starchy vegetables such as potatoes, corn, and peas) contain 15 grams of carbohydrate per choice.
- Foods on the **Nonstarchy Vegetables** list (such as green beans, tomatoes, and carrots) contain 5 grams of carbohydrate per choice.
- Foods on the **Protein** and **Fats** lists usually do not contain carbohydrate (except for plant-based protein foods such as beans and lentils). Most of the foods on the **Protein** list also contain fat.
- Some foods have so little carbohydrate and so few calories that they are considered "free," when eaten in small amounts. You can find these foods on the **Free Foods** list.
- The **Sweets, Desserts, and Other Carbohydrates** list, **Combination Foods** list (such as casseroles), and **Fast Foods** list include foods that have different amounts of carbohydrate and calories.
- Drinks on the **Alcohol** list contain calories, and some contain carbohydrate.

The Food Lists

The following chart shows the amount of nutrients in 1 choice from each list.

Food List	Carbohydrate (grams)	Protein (grams)	Fat (grams)	Calories
Carbohydrates				
Starch: breads; cereals; grains and pasta; starchy vegetables; crackers and snacks; and beans, peas, and lentils	15	3	1	80
Fruits	15	—	—	60
Milk and Milk Substitutes				
Fat-free, low-fat (1%)	12	8	0–3	100
Reduced-fat (2%)	12	8	5	120
Whole	12	8	8	160
Nonstarchy Vegetables	5	2	—	25
Sweets, Desserts, and Other Carbohydrates	15	varies	varies	varies
Proteins				
Lean	—	7	2	45
Medium-fat	—	7	5	75
High-fat	—	7	8	100
Plant-based	varies	7	varies	varies
Fats	—	—	5	45
Alcohol (1 alcohol equivalent)	varies	—	—	100

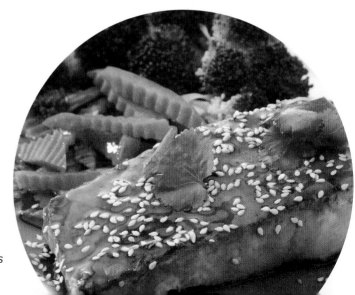

Other Features of *Choose Your Foods*

Other helpful features in this booklet include the following:

- **Reading Food Labels:** Nutrition Facts panels on labels are an important part of healthy eating. Each food list in this booklet shows average nutrient and calorie values, but these values aren't exact for specific foods. The information on the Nutrition Facts panel will give you the specific nutrient and calorie values you need to create a more accurate Eating Plan. (See page 56.)
- **Symbols:** The following symbols are used throughout this booklet to let you know which foods are good sources of fiber, which have extra fat, and which are high in sodium.

  ✓ **A good source of fiber** = More than 3 grams of dietary fiber per choice.

  ! **Extra fat** = A food with extra fat.

  !! **Added fat** = A food with two extra fat choices or a food prepared with added fat.

  ⬚ **High in sodium** = 480 milligrams or more of sodium per choice. (For foods listed as a main dish/meal on the **Combination Foods** and **Fast Foods** lists only, the ⬚ represents more than 600 milligrams of sodium per choice.) Eating less salt (sodium) is good for almost everyone, not just people with diabetes. High blood pressure can get worse if you eat too much sodium (salt and salty foods). When possible, use less salt in cooking and at the table. Snack foods, processed foods, canned soups, frozen meals and desserts, and restaurant foods all tend to be high in sodium.

- **Glossary:** You can look up diabetes-related words on pages 58–60.
- **Index:** If you are looking for a certain food or drink, look it up on pages 61–64.

Get Started

Your RDN will help you learn how to use the food lists in this booklet and improve your eating and physical activity habits. Together, you can also adjust your Eating Plan when your lifestyle or activity levels change. For example, you can change your Eating Plan to fit your work, school, vacation, or travel schedule.

Your RDN will also help you know when to check your blood glucose levels and what the numbers mean. By checking your blood glucose levels, you learn how different foods affect your blood glucose and you can figure out when you need to make changes in your Eating Plan or diabetes management plan. As you develop careful eating habits and control your blood glucose levels, you will feel better and be healthier, too.

Measurement Abbreviations
Tbsp = tablespoon
tsp = teaspoon
oz = ounce
fl oz = fluid ounce
lb = pound

Get Moving

Physical activity improves blood glucose control, reduces other health risks, and helps with weight management. Here are some tips to help you get started:

- Choose an activity you enjoy. Many people enjoy walking because it is easy to do and is free.
- Start with a daily goal of 5 to 10 minutes of physical activity, such as walking at a pace and distance that feels comfortable. Work up to at least 30 minutes a day, five times a week.
- Also include strength training for muscles at least twice a week in your physical activity plan.
- Wear comfortable shoes with good traction and shock absorption.
- Build exercise into your everyday activities. Take the stairs instead of the elevator. Park your car farther away from the office or store.
- Put extra effort into housework and chores, such as washing windows, scrubbing floors, vacuuming, and raking the yard.
- Short amounts of activity count. Three 10-minute walks add up to 30 minutes a day.
- Have backup plans for bad weather. Walk at the mall or find indoor activities you enjoy, such as walking on a treadmill or following a workout video or fitness TV show.

Breads, cereals, grains (including pasta and rice), starchy vegetables, crackers and snacks, and beans, peas, and lentils are starches. In general, **1 starch choice** is:

- ½ cup of cooked cereal, grain, or starchy vegetable
- ⅓ cup of cooked rice or pasta
- 1 oz of a bread product, such as 1 slice of bread
- ¾ to 1 oz of most snack foods (some snack foods may also have extra fat)

Nutrition Tips

- A choice on the **Starch** list has 15 grams of carbohydrate, 3 grams of protein, 1 gram of fat, and 80 calories.
- For health benefits, at least half of your servings of grains each day should be whole grains (see page 10 for more about whole grains).

Selection Tips

- Choose starches that are low in fat as often as possible.
- Starchy vegetables, baked goods, and grains that are prepared with fat count as 1 starch choice and 1 fat choice.
- For many starchy foods (bagels, muffins, dinner rolls, buns), a general rule of thumb is 1 oz equals 1 choice. Because of their large size, some foods have more carbohydrate and calories than you might think. For example, a large bagel may weigh 4 oz and equal 4 starch choices.
- For information about a specific food, read the Nutrition Facts panel on its food label.

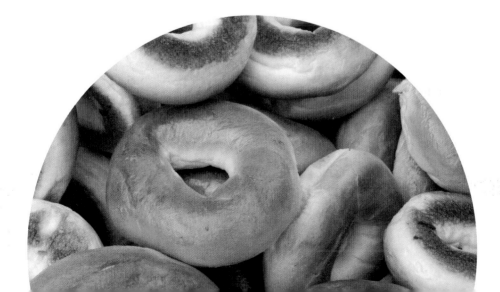

Gluten-Free Foods

Gluten is a protein in wheat, rye, and barley. If you cannot eat foods that contain gluten, always read food labels carefully.

- Foods that are labeled "gluten-free" can be included in your Eating Plan.
- For foods not labeled gluten-free, read the ingredients list. Do **not** eat foods that list wheat, barley, rye, malt, brewer's yeast, or regular oats.

When following a gluten-free diet, you can eat many starch foods, including:

- Baked goods, cereals, pasta, and other foods made with naturally gluten-free grains, such as rice or quinoa, instead of wheat, rye, or barley (**Note:** When choosing foods made with naturally gluten-free grains and flours, it is best to select products that are labeled gluten-free. The ingredients in products without the gluten-free label may have come into contact with grains that contain gluten.)
- Starchy vegetables, such as corn and potatoes
- Legumes, such as beans, peas, and lentils

You may also be able to eat oats and oat products that are labeled gluten-free. (Do **not** eat oats that are not labeled gluten-free. They may have come into contact with gluten.) Talk to your RDN or doctor about how many servings of gluten-free oats you can eat daily.

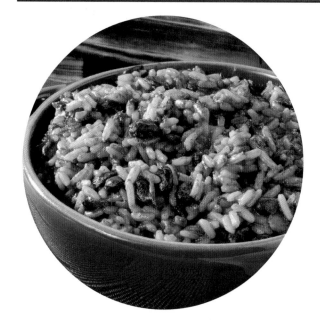

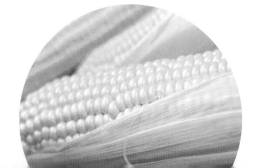

Choose Your Foods: Food Lists for Diabetes

One starch choice has 15 grams of carbohydrate, 3 grams of protein, 1 gram of fat, and 80 calories.

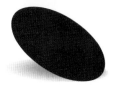

Bread

Food	Serving Size
Bagel	¼ large bagel (1 oz)
! Biscuit	1 biscuit (2½ inches across)
Breads, loaf-type	
white, whole-grain, French, Italian, pumpernickel, rye, sourdough, unfrosted raisin or cinnamon	1 slice (1 oz)
✓ reduced-calorie, light	2 slices (1½ oz)
Breads, flat-type (flatbreads)	
chapatti	1 oz
ciabatta	1 oz
naan	3¼-inch square (1 oz)
pita (6 inches across)	½ pita
roti	1 oz
✓ sandwich flat buns, whole-wheat	1 bun, including top and bottom (1½ oz)
! taco shell	2 taco shells (each 5 inches across)
tortilla, corn	1 small tortilla (6 inches across)
tortilla, flour (white or whole-wheat)	1 small tortilla (6 inches across) or ⅓ large tortilla (10 inches across)
Cornbread	1¾-inch cube (1½ oz)
English muffin	½ muffin
Hot dog bun or hamburger bun	½ bun (¾ oz)
Pancake	1 pancake (4 inches across, ¼ inch thick)
Roll, plain	1 small roll (1 oz)
! Stuffing, bread	⅓ cup
Waffle	1 waffle (4-inch square or 4 inches across)

 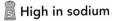

Cereals

Food	Serving Size
✓ Bran cereal (twigs, buds, or flakes)	½ cup
Cooked cereals (oats, oatmeal)	½ cup
Granola cereal	¼ cup
Grits, cooked	½ cup
Muesli	¼ cup
Puffed cereal	1½ cups
Shredded wheat, plain	½ cup
Sugar-coated cereal	½ cup
Unsweetened, ready-to-eat cereal	¾ cup

Whole Grains

Whole grains and whole-grain products contain the entire grain seed of a plant. They are rich in fiber, vitamins, and minerals. Here are some tips for including more whole grains in your diet:

- Choose whole-grain foods more often. Whole-grain foods include whole-wheat flour, whole oats/oatmeal, whole-grain cornmeal, popcorn, buckwheat, buckwheat flour, whole rye, whole-grain barley, brown rice, wild rice, bulgur, millet, quinoa, and sorghum.
- Read food labels carefully. If a product label says "100% whole grain," it must contain at least 16 grams of whole grain per serving.
- Add several tablespoons of cooked grains to stews, soups, and vegetable salads.
- Monitor your blood glucose level carefully to find out the effect that whole grains have on you.

Choose Your Foods: Food Lists for Diabetes

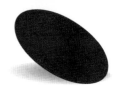

One starch choice has 15 grams of carbohydrate, 3 grams of protein, 1 gram of fat, and 80 calories.

Grains (Including Pasta and Rice)

Unless otherwise indicated, serving sizes listed are for cooked grains.

Food	Serving Size
Barley	⅓ cup
Bran, dry	
✔ oat	¼ cup
✔ wheat	½ cup
✔ Bulgur	½ cup
Couscous	⅓ cup
Kasha	½ cup
Millet	⅓ cup
Pasta, white or whole-wheat (all shapes and sizes)	⅓ cup
Polenta	⅓ cup
Quinoa, all colors	⅓ cup
Rice, white, brown, and other colors and types	⅓ cup
Tabbouleh (tabouli), prepared	½ cup
Wheat germ, dry	3 Tbsp
Wild rice	½ cup

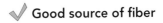 ✔ **Good source of fiber** 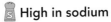 ! **Extra fat** 🧂 **High in sodium**

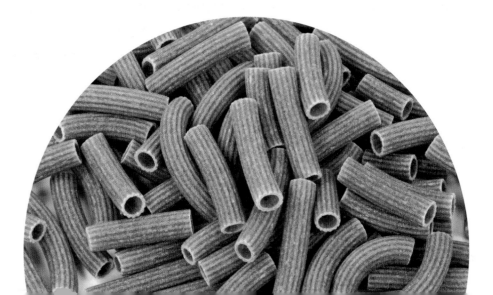

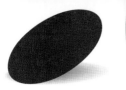

Starch

Starchy Vegetables

All of the serving sizes for starchy vegetables on this list are for cooked vegetables.

Food	Serving Size
Breadfruit	¼ cup
Cassava or dasheen	⅓ cup
Corn	½ cup
on cob	4- to 4½-inch piece (½ large cob)
✓ Hominy	¾ cup
✓ Mixed vegetables with corn or peas	1 cup
Marinara, pasta, or spaghetti sauce	½ cup
✓ Parsnips	½ cup
✓ Peas, green	½ cup
Plantain	⅓ cup
Potato	
baked with skin	¼ large potato (3 oz)
boiled, all kinds	½ cup or ½ medium potato (3 oz)
! mashed, with milk and fat	½ cup
French-fried (oven-baked)*	1 cup (2 oz)
✓ Pumpkin puree, canned, no sugar added	¾ cup
✓ Squash, winter (acorn, butternut)	1 cup
✓ Succotash	½ cup
Yam or sweet potato, plain	½ cup (3½ oz)

*Note: Restaurant-style French fries are on the **Fast Foods** list, page 54.

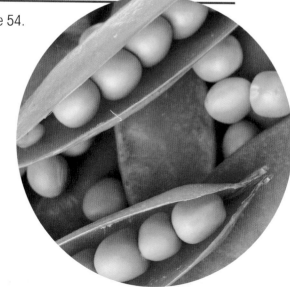

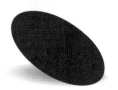

One starch choice has 15 grams of carbohydrate, 3 grams of protein, 1 gram of fat, and 80 calories.

Crackers and Snacks

Note: Some snacks are high in fat. Always check food labels.

Food	Serving Size
Crackers	
✓ animal	8 crackers
✓ crispbread	2 to 5 pieces (¾ oz)
graham, 2½-inch square	3 squares
nut and rice	10 crackers
oyster	20 crackers
❗ round, butter-type	6 crackers
saltine-type	6 crackers
❗ sandwich-style, cheese or peanut butter filling	3 crackers
whole-wheat, baked	5 regular 1½-inch squares or 10 thins (¾ oz)
Granola or snack bar	1 bar (¾ oz)
Matzoh, all shapes and sizes	¾ oz
Melba toast	4 pieces (each about 2 by 4 inches)
Popcorn	
✓ no fat added	3 cups
❗❗ with butter added	3 cups
Pretzels	¾ oz
Rice cakes	2 cakes (4 inches across)
Snack chips	
baked (potato, pita)	about 8 chips (¾ oz)
❗❗ regular (tortilla, potato)	about 13 chips (1 oz)

❗ count as 1 starch choice + 1 fat choice (1 starch choice plus 5 grams of fat)

❗❗ count as 1 starch choice + 2 fat choices (1 starch choice plus 10 grams of fat)

Note: For other snacks, see the **Sweets, Desserts, and Other Carbohydrates** list, page 25.

TIP An open handful is equal to about 1 cup or 1 to 2 oz of snack food.

✓ Good source of fiber   ❗ Extra fat   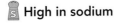 High in sodium

Beans, Peas, and Lentils

The choices on this list count as 1 starch choice + 1 lean protein choice.

	Food	Serving Size
✓	Baked beans, canned	⅓ cup
✓	Beans (black, garbanzo, kidney, lima, navy, pinto, white), cooked or canned, drained and rinsed	½ cup
✓	Lentils (any color), cooked	½ cup
✓	Peas (black-eyed and split), cooked or canned, drained and rinsed	½ cup
⑤ ✓	Refried beans, canned	½ cup

Note: Beans, lentils, and peas are also found on the **Protein** list, page 36.

✓ **Good source of fiber**　　❗ **Extra fat**　　⑤ **High in sodium**

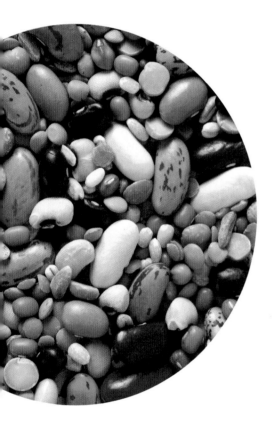

> **TIP** Canned beans, lentils, and peas can be high in sodium (salt). Draining and rinsing them reduces the sodium content by at least 40%.

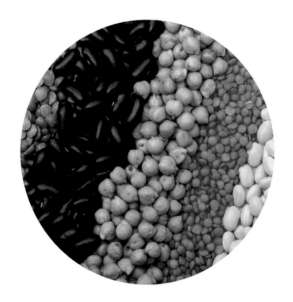

Fruits

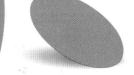

Fresh, frozen, canned, and dried fruits and fruit juices are on this list. In general, **1 fruit choice** is:

- ½ cup of canned or frozen fruit
- 1 small fresh fruit (¾ to 1 cup)
- ½ cup of unsweetened fruit juice
- 2 tablespoons of dried fruit

Nutrition Tips

- A choice on the **Fruits** list has 15 grams of carbohydrate, 0 grams of protein, 0 grams of fat, and 60 calories.
- Fresh, frozen, and dried fruits are good sources of fiber. Fruit juices contain very little fiber. Choose fruits instead of juices whenever possible.
- Citrus fruits, berries, and melons are good sources of vitamin C.

Selection Tips

- Some fruits on the list are measured by weight. The weights listed include skin, core, seeds, and rind. Use a food scale to weigh fresh fruits and figure out how many choices you are eating.
- Read the Nutrition Facts panel on food labels of packaged fruits and juices. If 1 serving has more than 15 grams of carbohydrate, you may need to adjust the size of the serving to fit with the choices in your Eating Plan.
- Serving sizes for canned fruits on the **Fruits** list are for the fruit and a small amount of juice (1 to 2 tablespoons).
- Food labels for fruits and fruit juices may contain the words "no sugar added" or "unsweetened." This means that no sugar, other than the sugar from the fruit itself, has been added. It does not mean the food contains no sugar.
- Fruit canned in extra-light syrup has the same amount of carbohydrate per serving as canned fruit labeled "no sugar added" or "juice pack." All canned fruits on the **Fruits** list are based on one of these three types of pack. Avoid fruit canned in heavy syrup.

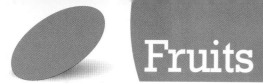

Fruits

The weights listed include skin, core, seeds, and rind.

Food	Serving Size
Apple, unpeeled	1 small apple (4 oz)
Apples, dried	4 rings
Applesauce, unsweetened	½ cup
Apricots	
canned	½ cup
dried	8 apricot halves
fresh	4 apricots (5½ oz total)
Banana	1 extra-small banana, about 4 inches long (4 oz)
✓ Blackberries	1 cup
Blueberries	¾ cup
Cantaloupe	1 cup diced
Cherries	
sweet, canned	½ cup
sweet, fresh	12 cherries (3½ oz)
Dates	3 small (deglet noor) dates or 1 large (medjool) date
Dried fruits (blueberries, cherries, cranberries, mixed fruit, raisins)	2 Tbsp
Figs	
dried	3 small figs
✓ fresh	1½ large or 2 medium figs (3½ oz total)
Fruit cocktail	½ cup
Grapefruit	
fresh	½ large grapefruit (5½ oz)
sections, canned	¾ cup
Grapes	17 small grapes (3 oz total)
✓ Guava	2 small guava (2½ oz total)

(continued on next page)

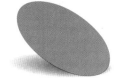

One fruit choice has 15 grams of carbohydrate and 60 calories.

Fruits (continued)

The weights listed include skin, core, seeds, and rind.

Food	Serving Size
Honeydew melon	1 cup diced
Kiwi	½ cup sliced
Loquat	¾ cup cubed
Mandarin oranges, canned	¾ cup
Mango	½ small mango (5½ oz) or ½ cup
Nectarine	1 medium nectarine (5½ oz)
✓ Orange	1 medium orange (6½ oz)
Papaya	½ papaya (8 oz) or 1 cup cubed
Peaches	
canned	½ cup
fresh	1 medium peach (6 oz)
Pears	
canned	½ cup
✓ fresh	½ large pear (4 oz)
Pineapple	
canned	½ cup
fresh	¾ cup
Plantain, extra-ripe (black), raw	¼ plantain (2¼ oz)
Plums	
canned	½ cup
dried (prunes)	3 prunes
fresh	2 small plums (5 oz total)
Pomegranate seeds (arils)	½ cup
✓ Raspberries	1 cup
✓ Strawberries	1¼ cup whole berries
Tangerine	1 large tangerine (6 oz)
Watermelon	1¼ cups diced

 ✓ Good source of fiber   ! Extra fat   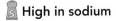 High in sodium

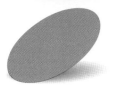

Fruits

Fruit Juice

Food	Serving Size
Apple juice/cider	½ cup
Fruit juice blends, 100% juice	⅓ cup
Grape juice	⅓ cup
Grapefruit juice	½ cup
Orange juice	½ cup
Pineapple juice	½ cup
Pomegranate juice	½ cup
Prune juice	⅓ cup

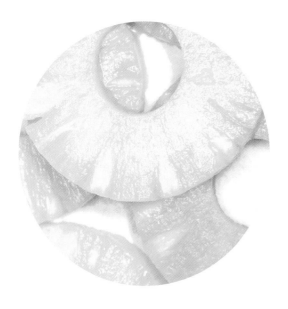

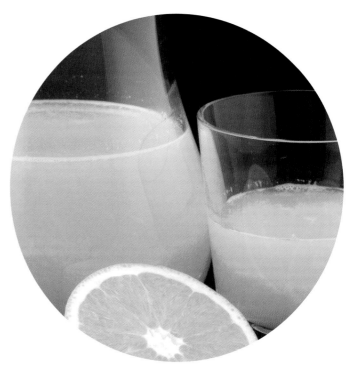

Milk and Milk Substitutes

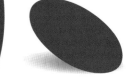

Different types of milk, milk products, and milk substitutes are included on this list. However, certain types of milk and milk-like products are found on other lists:

- Cheeses are on the **Protein** list (because they are rich in protein and have very little carbohydrate).
- Butter, cream, coffee creamers, and unsweetened nut milks are on the **Fats** list.
- Ice cream and frozen yogurt are on the **Sweets, Desserts, and Other Carbohydrates** list.

Nutrition Tips

- Milk and yogurt are good sources of calcium and protein.
- Greek yogurt contains more protein and less carbohydrate than most other yogurts.
- Types of milk and yogurt that are high in fat (2% or whole milk) have more saturated fat, cholesterol, and calories than low-fat or fat-free milk and yogurt.
- Children older than 2 years and adults should choose lower-fat varieties of milk and milk products, such as fat-free (skim) or low-fat (1%) milk or low-fat or nonfat yogurt.

Selection Tip

- 1 cup equals 8 fluid oz or ½ pint.

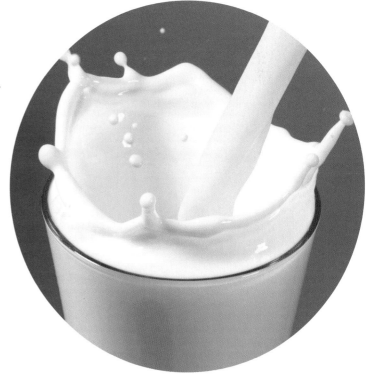

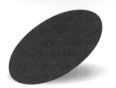

Milk and Milk Substitutes

One milk choice has 12 grams of carbohydrate and 8 grams of protein and:

- One fat-free (skim) or low-fat (1%) milk choice has 0–3 grams of fat and 100 calories per serving.
- One reduced-fat (2%) milk choice has 5 grams of fat and 120 calories per serving.
- One whole milk choice has 8 grams of fat and 160 calories per serving.

Milk and Yogurts

Food	Serving Size	Choices per Serving
Fat-free (skim) or low-fat (1%)		
milk, buttermilk, acidophilus milk, lactose-free milk	1 cup	1 fat-free milk
evaporated milk	½ cup	1 fat-free milk
yogurt, plain or Greek; may be sweetened with an artificial sweetener	⅔ cup (6 oz)	1 fat-free milk
Chocolate milk	1 cup	1 fat-free milk + 1 carbohydrate
Reduced-fat (2%)		
milk, acidophilus milk, kefir, lactose-free milk	1 cup	1 reduced-fat milk
yogurt, plain	⅔ cup (6 oz)	1 reduced-fat milk
Whole		
milk, buttermilk, goat's milk	1 cup	1 whole milk
evaporated milk	½ cup	1 whole milk
yogurt, plain	1 cup (8 oz)	1 whole milk
chocolate milk	1 cup	1 whole milk + 1 carbohydrate

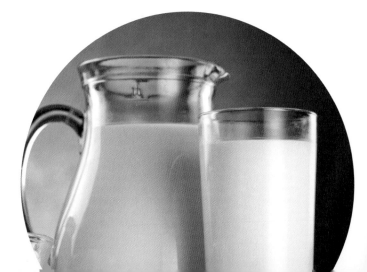

Choose Your Foods: Food Lists for Diabetes

One carbohydrate choice has 15 grams of carbohydrate and about 70 calories. One fat choice has 5 grams of fat and 45 calories.

Other Milk Foods and Milk Substitutes

Food	Serving Size	Choices per Serving
Eggnog		
fat-free	⅓ cup	1 carbohydrate
low-fat	⅓ cup	1 carbohydrate + ½ fat
whole milk	⅓ cup	1 carbohydrate + 1 fat
Rice drink		
plain, fat-free	1 cup	1 carbohydrate
flavored, low-fat	1 cup	2 carbohydrates
Soy milk		
light or low-fat, plain	1 cup	½ carbohydrate + ½ fat
regular, plain	1 cup	½ carbohydrate + 1 fat
Yogurt with fruit, low-fat	⅔ cup (6 oz)	1 fat-free milk + 1 carbohydrate

Note: Unsweetened nut milks (such as almond milk and coconut milk) are on the **Fats** list, page 39.

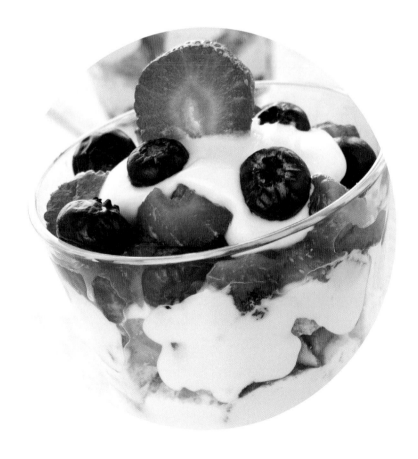

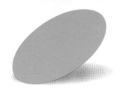

Nonstarchy Vegetables

Vegetables that contain a small amount of carbohydrate and few calories are on this list. (Vegetables that contain higher amounts of carbohydrate and calories can be found on the **Starch** list.) In general, **1 nonstarchy vegetable choice** is:

- ½ cup of cooked vegetables or vegetable juice
- 1 cup of raw vegetables

If you eat 3 cups or more of raw vegetables or 1½ cups or more of cooked nonstarchy vegetables in a meal, count them as 1 carbohydrate choice.

Nutrition Tips

- A choice on the **Nonstarchy Vegetables** list has 5 grams of carbohydrate, 2 grams of protein, 0 grams of fat, and 25 calories.
- Nonstarchy and starchy vegetables both contain important nutrients. Try to choose a variety of vegetables and **eat at least 2 to 3 nonstarchy vegetable choices daily.**
- Fresh, plain vegetables have no added salt. When choosing canned or frozen vegetables, read food labels and look for low-sodium or no-salt-added varieties. If these are not available, you can drain and rinse canned vegetables to reduce their sodium content.
- Read the Nutrition Facts panel on labels for canned and frozen vegetables. In addition to sodium, some products have added fats and sauces, which increase the calories and carbohydrate.
- Read labels on canned vegetable juices, too, and choose no-salt-added or low-sodium products.
- Vegetables that are deep in color, such as dark green or dark yellow vegetables, offer many nutritional benefits. Good daily choices include spinach, kale, broccoli, romaine, carrots, and peppers.
- Good sources of vitamin C include broccoli, brussels sprouts, cauliflower, greens, peppers, spinach, and tomatoes.
- Vegetables from the cruciferous family are rich in nutrients and offer health benefits. Eat them several times each week. Choices include bok choy, broccoli, brussels sprouts, cabbage, cauliflower, collards, kale, kohlrabi, radishes, rutabaga, and turnips.
- Many vegetables are a good source of dietary fiber.
- Raw sprouts, such as alfalfa or bean sprouts, may cause foodborne illness. For this reason, you should not eat raw sprouts.

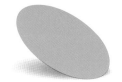

One nonstarchy vegetable choice (½ cup cooked or 1 cup raw) has 5 grams of carbohydrate, 2 grams of protein, 0 grams of fat, and 25 calories.

Selection Tips

- One cup of raw vegetables is a portion about the size of a baseball or your fist.
- The tomato sauce referred to in this list is different from spaghetti/pasta sauce, which usually contains added sugar and is on the **Starchy Vegetables** list.

Eating More Vegetables

Vegetables are an important part of any healthy Eating Plan. Here are some tips for adding nonstarchy vegetables to your plan:

- Store vegetables in a visible place in your refrigerator instead of hidden in a produce drawer. When you see them, you are more likely to eat them.
- Wash and pre-cut raw vegetables, such as carrots, asparagus, broccoli, radishes, cauliflower, celery, bell peppers, and cherry tomatoes, so they are ready to use for meals and snacks.
- For convenience, buy premixed, bagged salads. (Avoid those with dressing packets or high-fat garnishes, such as croutons and bacon bits.)
- Enjoy sandwiches made with generous amounts of nonstarchy vegetables, such as lettuce, spinach leaves, chopped cabbage, onion, cucumbers, tomatoes, and bell peppers.
- Stir raw or lightly cooked vegetables into pasta, rice, and omelets.
- Add chopped vegetables to soups or stews.
- Add finely chopped vegetables, such as carrots, onions, cooked eggplant, squash, or spinach, to pasta sauce.
- Keep a single-serving can of vegetable or tomato juice (low-sodium or no-added-salt) in your bookbag, briefcase, or purse for a quick snack.
- Top a baked potato with salsa or stir-fried vegetables.

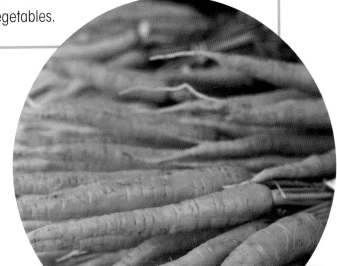

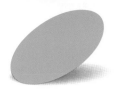

Nonstarchy Vegetables

Nonstarchy Vegetables

Amaranth leaves (Chinese spinach)

Artichoke

Artichoke hearts (no oil)

Asparagus

Baby corn

Bamboo shoots

Bean sprouts (alfalfa, mung, soybean)

Beans (green, wax, Italian, yard-long beans)

Beets

Broccoli

Broccoli slaw, packaged, no dressing

✓ Brussels sprouts

Cabbage (green, red, bok choy, Chinese)

✓ Carrots

Cauliflower

Celery

Chayote

Coleslaw, packaged, no dressing

Cucumber

Daikon

Eggplant

Fennel

Gourds (bitter, bottle, luffa, bitter melon)

Green onions or scallions

Greens (collard, dandelion, mustard, purslane, turnip)

Hearts of palm

✓ Jicama

Kale

Kohlrabi

Leeks

Mixed vegetables (without starchy vegetables, legumes, or pasta)

Mushrooms, all kinds, fresh

Okra

Onions

Pea pods

Peppers (all varieties)

Radishes

Rutabaga

⑤ Sauerkraut, drained and rinsed

Spinach

Squash, summer varieties (yellow, pattypan, crookneck, zucchini)

Sugar snap peas

Swiss chard

Tomato

Tomatoes, canned

⑤ Tomato sauce (unsweetened)

Tomato/vegetable juice

Turnips

Water chestnuts

Note: Salad greens (like arugula, chicory, endive, escarole, lettuce, radicchio, romaine, and watercress) are on the **Free Foods** list, page 43.

 Good source of fiber **Extra fat** ⑤ **High in sodium**

Choose Your Foods: Food Lists for Diabetes

Sweets, Desserts, and Other Carbohydrates

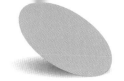

Foods on this list have added sugars or fat. However, you can substitute food choices from this list for other carbohydrate-containing foods.

Nutrition Tips

- A carbohydrate choice in this list has 15 grams of carbohydrate and about 70 calories.
- Choose foods from this list less often. They do not have as many vitamins or minerals or as much fiber as the choices on the **Starch, Fruits,** and **Milk and Milk Substitutes** lists. Balance your meal by eating foods from other food lists to get the nutrients your body needs.
- Many of the foods on the **Sweets, Desserts, and Other Carbohydrates** list contain more than a single choice of carbohydrate. Some will also count as one or more fat choices.
- The serving sizes for foods on this list are small because these foods are high in calories.

Selection Tips

- Read the Nutrition Facts panel on the food label to find the serving size and nutrient information. Remember: The label serving size may be different from the serving size used in this food list.
- Many sugar-free, fat-free, or reduced-fat products are made with ingredients that contain carbohydrate. These types of food often have the same amount of carbohydrate as the regular foods they are replacing. Talk with your RDN to find out how to fit these foods into your Eating Plan.

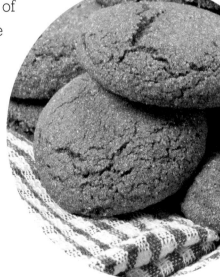

Common Measurements	
Dry	**Liquid**
3 tsp = 1 Tbsp	4 Tbsp = ¼ cup
4 oz = ½ cup	8 oz = 1 cup or
8 oz = 1 cup	½ pint

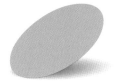

Sweets, Desserts, and Other Carbohydrates

Beverages, Soda, and Sports Drinks

Food	Serving Size	Choices per Serving
Cranberry juice cocktail	½ cup	1 carbohydrate
Fruit drink or lemonade	1 cup (8 oz)	2 carbohydrates
Hot chocolate, regular	1 envelope (2 Tbsp or ¾ oz) added to 8 oz water	1 carbohydrate
Soft drink (soda), regular	1 can (12 oz)	2½ carbohydrates
Sports drink (fluid replacement type)	1 cup (8 oz)	1 carbohydrate

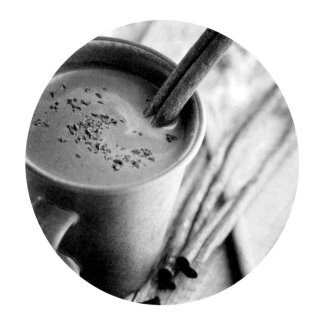

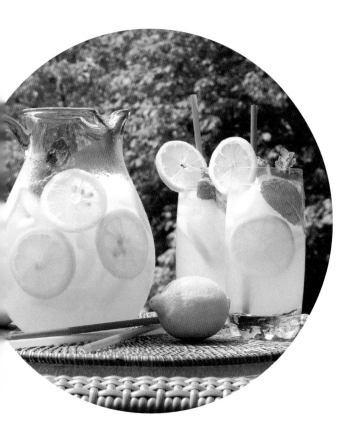

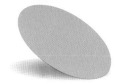

Brownies, Cake, Cookies, Gelatin, Pie, and Pudding

Food	Serving Size	Choices per Serving
Biscotti	1 oz	1 carbohydrate + 1 fat
Brownie, small, unfrosted	1¼-inch square, ⅞-inch high (about 1 oz)	1 carbohydrate + 1 fat
Cake		
angel food, unfrosted	¹⁄₁₂ of cake (about 2 oz)	2 carbohydrates
frosted	2-inch square (about 2 oz)	2 carbohydrates + 1 fat
unfrosted	2-inch square (about 1 oz)	1 carbohydrate + 1 fat
Cookies		
100-calorie pack	1 oz	1 carbohydrate + ½ fat
chocolate chip cookies	2 cookies, 2¼ inches across	1 carbohydrate + 2 fats
gingersnaps	3 small cookies, 1½ inches across	1 carbohydrate
large cookie	1 cookie, 6 inches across (about 3 oz)	4 carbohydrates + 3 fats
sandwich cookies with crème filling	2 small cookies (about ⅔ oz)	1 carbohydrate + 1 fat
sugar-free cookies	1 large or 3 small cookies (¾ to 1 oz)	1 carbohydrate + 1 to 2 fats
vanilla wafer	5 cookies	1 carbohydrate + 1 fat
Cupcake, frosted	1 small cupcake (about 1¾ oz)	2 carbohydrates + 1 to 1½ fats
Flan	½ cup	2½ carbohydrates + 1 fat
Fruit cobbler	½ cup (3½ oz)	3 carbohydrates + 1 fat
Gelatin, regular	½ cup	1 carbohydrate
Pie		
commercially prepared fruit, 2 crusts	⅙ of 8-inch pie	3 carbohydrates + 2 fats
pumpkin or custard	⅛ of 8-inch pie	1½ carbohydrates + 1½ fats
Pudding		
regular (made with reduced-fat milk)	½ cup	2 carbohydrates
sugar-free or sugar- and fat-free (made with fat-free milk)	½ cup	1 carbohydrate

Sweets, Desserts, and Other Carbohydrates

Candy, Spreads, Sweets, Sweeteners, Syrups, and Toppings

Food	Serving Size	Choices per Serving
Blended sweeteners (mixtures of artificial sweeteners and sugar)	1½ Tbsp	1 carbohydrate
Candy		
chocolate, dark or milk type	1 oz	1 carbohydrate + 2 fats
chocolate "kisses"	5 pieces	1 carbohydrate + 1 fat
hard	3 pieces	1 carbohydrate
Coffee creamer, nondairy type		
powdered, flavored	4 tsp	½ carbohydrate + ½ fat
liquid, flavored	2 Tbsp	1 carbohydrate
Fruit snacks, chewy (pureed fruit concentrate)	1 roll (¾ oz)	1 carbohydrate
Fruit spreads, 100% fruit	1½ Tbsp	1 carbohydrate
Honey	1 Tbsp	1 carbohydrate
Jam or jelly, regular	1 Tbsp	1 carbohydrate
Sugar	1 Tbsp	1 carbohydrate
Syrup		
chocolate	2 Tbsp	2 carbohydrates
light (pancake-type)	2 Tbsp	1 carbohydrate
regular (pancake-type)	1 Tbsp	1 carbohydrate

Condiments and Sauces

Food	Serving Size	Choices per Serving
Barbecue sauce	3 Tbsp	1 carbohydrate
Cranberry sauce, jellied	¼ cup	1½ carbohydrates
Curry sauce	1 oz	1 carbohydrate + 1 fat
Gravy, canned or bottled	½ cup	½ carbohydrate + ½ fat
Hoisin sauce	1 Tbsp	½ carbohydrate
Marinade	1 Tbsp	½ carbohydrate
Plum sauce	1 Tbsp	½ carbohydrate
Salad dressing, fat-free, cream-based	3 Tbsp	1 carbohydrate
Sweet-and-sour sauce	3 Tbsp	1 carbohydrate

Note: You can also check the **Fats** list and **Free Foods** list for other condiments.

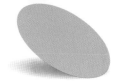

Doughnuts, Muffins, Pastries, and Sweet Breads

Food	Serving Size	Choices per Serving
Banana nut bread	1-inch slice (2 oz)	2 carbohydrates + 1 fat
Doughnut		
cake, plain	1 medium doughnut (1½ oz)	1½ carbohydrates + 2 fats
hole	2 holes (1 oz)	1 carbohydrate + 1 fat
yeast-type, glazed	1 doughnut, 3¾ inches across (2 oz)	2 carbohydrates + 2 fats
Muffin		
regular	1 muffin (4 oz)	4 carbohydrates + 2½ fats
lower-fat	1 muffin (4 oz)	4 carbohydrates + ½ fat
Scone	1 scone (4 oz)	4 carbohydrates + 3 fats
Sweet roll or Danish	1 pastry (2½ oz)	2½ carbohydrates + 2 fats

Frozen Bars, Frozen Desserts, Frozen Yogurt, and Ice Cream

Food	Serving Size	Choices per Serving
Frozen pops	1	½ carbohydrate
Fruit juice bars, frozen, 100% juice	1 bar (3 oz)	1 carbohydrate
Ice cream		
fat-free	½ cup	1½ carbohydrates
light	½ cup	1 carbohydrate + 1 fat
no-sugar-added	½ cup	1 carbohydrate + 1 fat
regular	½ cup	1 carbohydrate + 2 fats
Sherbet, sorbet	½ cup	2 carbohydrates
Yogurt, frozen		
fat-free	⅓ cup	1 carbohydrate
regular	½ cup	1 carbohydrate + 0 to 1 fat
Greek, lower-fat or fat-free	½ cup	1½ carbohydrates

✓ Good source of fiber   ! Extra fat   🧂 High in sodium

29

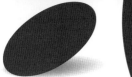

Protein

Meat, fish, poultry, cheese, eggs, and plant-based foods are all sources of protein and have varying amounts of fat. Foods from this list are divided into four groups based on the amount of fat they contain. These groups are lean protein, medium-fat protein, high-fat protein, and plant-based protein. The following chart shows you what one protein choice includes.

	Carbohydrate (grams)	Protein (grams)	Fat (grams)	Calories
Lean protein	—	7	2	45
Medium-fat protein	—	7	5	75
High-fat protein	—	7	8	100
Plant-based protein	varies	7	varies	varies

Some meals may have more than 1 protein choice. For example, a breakfast sandwich may be made with 1 ounce of cheese and 1 egg. Since 1 ounce of cheese counts as 1 protein choice and 1 egg counts as 1 protein choice, this meal would contain 2 protein choices. As another example, if you eat 3 ounces of cooked chicken at dinner, this portion would equal 3 protein choices because each ounce counts as 1 protein choice. Some snacks may also contain protein. Talk to your RDN to find out how many protein choices to eat each day.

Nutrition Tips

- Many types of fish (halibut, herring, mackerel, salmon, sardines, trout, and tuna) are rich in omega-3 fats, which may help reduce risk for heart disease. Choose fish (not commercially fried fish fillets) two or more times each week.
- Whenever possible, choose lean meats because they have less saturated fat and cholesterol than medium-fat and high-fat meats.
  - Select grades of meat are the leanest.
  - Choice grades have a moderate amount of fat.
  - Prime cuts of meat have the highest amount of fat.

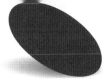

One lean protein choice has 0 grams of carbohydrate, 7 grams of protein, 2 grams of fat, and 45 calories.

Selection Tips

- Read labels to find foods low in fat and cholesterol. Aim for 5 grams of fat or less per protein choice (serving size, usually 1 oz).
- Read labels to find "hidden" carbohydrate. For example, meatless or vegetable burgers may contain quite a bit of carbohydrate. Check the Nutrition Facts panel on the label to see if the total carbohydrate in 1 serving is close to 15 grams. If it is close to 15 grams, count it as 1 carbohydrate choice and 1 protein choice.
- Processed meats, such as hot dogs and sausages, are often high in fat and sodium. Look for lower-fat and lower-sodium versions.

Portion Sizes

Portion size is an important part of meal planning. The **Protein** list is based on cooked weight (for example, 4 oz of raw meat is equal to 3 oz of cooked meat) after bone and fat have been removed. Try using the following comparisons to help estimate portion sizes:

- 1 oz cooked meat, poultry, or fish is about the size of a small matchbox.
- 3 oz cooked meat, poultry, or fish is about the size of a deck of playing cards.
- 2 tablespoons peanut butter is about the size of a golf ball.
- The palm of a woman's hand is about the size of 3 to 4 oz of cooked, boneless meat. The palm of a man's hand is about the size of 4 to 6 oz of cooked, boneless meat.
- 1 oz cheese is about the size of 4 dice.

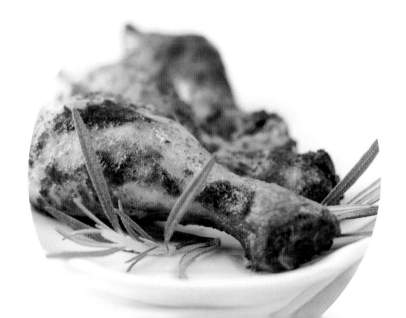

Cooking Tips

- Bake, poach, steam, or boil instead of frying.
- Roast, broil, or grill meat on a rack to drain off fat during cooking.
- Trim off visible fat or skin.
- Use a nonstick spray or a nonstick pan to brown or fry foods.
- Meat or fish that is breaded with cornmeal, flour, or dried bread crumbs contains carbohydrate. Count 3 tablespoons of one of these dry starches as 15 grams of carbohydrate.

Ground Beef Labeling

Some ground beef is labeled by cut, and others are labeled by lean-to-fat percentages. Ground beef is highest in fat, about 30% fat, followed by ground chuck, about 20% fat. Ground round and ground sirloin each have about 11% fat.

However, the grade of meat stated on the label does not always indicate how lean the meat is. All packaged ground beef has some fat. Look for lean ground beef choices such as 90% lean/10% fat.

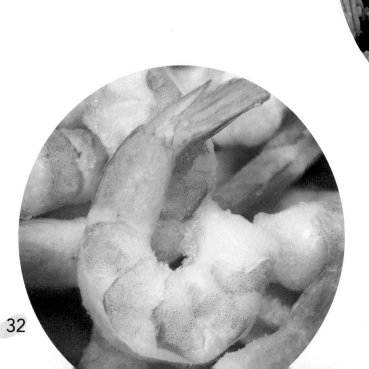

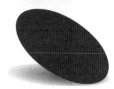

One lean protein choice has 0 grams of carbohydrate, 7 grams of protein, 2 grams of fat, and 45 calories.

Lean Protein

Note: 1 oz is usually the serving size for meat, fish, poultry, or hard cheeses.

	Food	Serving Size
	Beef: ground (90% or higher lean/10% or lower fat); select or choice grades trimmed of fat: roast (chuck, round, rump, sirloin), steak (cubed, flank, porterhouse, T-bone), tenderloin	1 oz
S	Beef jerky	½ oz
	Cheeses with 3 grams of fat or less per oz	1 oz
	Curd-style cheeses: cottage-type (all kinds); ricotta (fat-free or light)	¼ cup (2 oz)
	Egg substitutes, plain	¼ cup
	Egg whites	2
	Fish	
	fresh or frozen, such as catfish, cod, flounder, haddock, halibut, orange roughy, tilapia, trout	1 oz
	salmon, fresh or canned	1 oz
	sardines, canned	2 small sardines
	tuna, fresh or canned in water or oil and drained	1 oz
S	smoked: herring or salmon (lox)	1 oz
	Game: buffalo, ostrich, rabbit, venison	1 oz
S	Hot dog with 3 grams of fat or less per oz Note: May contain carbohydrate.	1 hot dog (1¾ oz)
	Lamb: chop, leg, or roast	1 oz
	Organ meats: heart, kidney, liver Note: May be high in cholesterol.	1 oz
	Oysters, fresh or frozen	6 medium oysters
	Pork, lean	
S	Canadian bacon	1 oz
S	ham	1 oz
	rib or loin chop/roast, tenderloin	1 oz
	Poultry, without skin: chicken; Cornish hen; domestic duck or goose (well-drained of fat); turkey; lean ground turkey or chicken	1 oz
S	Processed sandwich meats with 3 grams of fat or less per oz: chipped beef, thin-sliced deli meats, turkey ham, turkey pastrami	1 oz
S	Sausage with 3 grams of fat or less per oz	1 oz
	Shellfish: clams, crab, imitation shellfish, lobster, scallops, shrimp	1 oz
	Veal: cutlet (no breading), loin chop, roast	1 oz

✔ **Good source of fiber** S **High in sodium** (based on the sodium content of a typical 3-oz
! **Extra fat** serving of meat, unless 1 oz or 2 oz is the normal serving size)

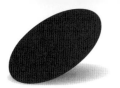

Protein

One medium-fat protein choice has 0 grams of carbohydrate, 7 grams of protein, 5 grams of fat, and 75 calories.

Medium-Fat Protein

Note: 1 oz is usually the serving size for meat, fish, poultry, or hard cheeses.

Food	Serving Size
Beef trimmed of visible fat: ground beef (85% or lower lean/15% or higher fat), corned beef, meatloaf, prime cuts of beef (rib roast), short ribs, tongue	1 oz
Cheeses with 4 to 7 grams of fat per oz: feta, mozzarella, pasteurized processed cheese spread, reduced-fat cheeses	1 oz
Cheese, ricotta (regular or part-skim)	¼ cup (2 oz)
Egg	1 egg
Fish: any fried	1 oz
Lamb: ground, rib roast	1 oz
Pork: cutlet, ground, shoulder roast	1 oz
Poultry with skin: chicken, dove, pheasant, turkey, wild duck, or goose; fried chicken	1 oz
Sausage with 4 to 7 grams of fat per oz	1 oz

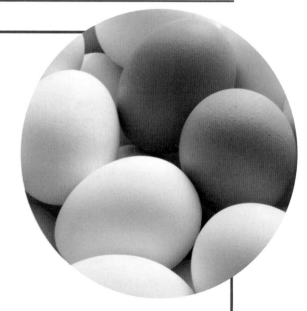

Smart Food Shopping

- Don't shop when you're hungry.
- Shop early in the day.
- Shop alone.
- Use a list.
- Shop the outer sections of the supermarket to select more fresh foods and fewer processed foods.
- Choose a variety of colorful fruits and vegetables.
- Go for whole grains.
- Be adventurous. Give new foods a try.
- Read food labels.
- Skip the "diabetic" food. There is no need for people with diabetes to eat "special" and usually more expensive foods.

Choose Your Foods: Food Lists for Diabetes

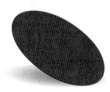

One high-fat protein choice has 0 grams of carbohydrate, 7 grams of protein, 8 grams of fat, and 100 calories.

High-Fat Protein

These foods are high in saturated fat, cholesterol, and calories and may raise blood cholesterol levels if eaten on a regular basis. Try to eat 3 or fewer choices from this group per week.

Note: 1 oz is usually the serving size for meat, fish, poultry, or hard cheeses.

Food	Serving Size
Bacon, pork	2 slices (1 oz each before cooking)
⬛ Bacon, turkey	3 slices (½ oz each before cooking)
Cheese, regular: American, blue-veined, brie, cheddar, hard goat, Monterey jack, Parmesan, queso, and Swiss	1 oz
! Hot dog: beef, pork, or combination	1 hot dog (10 hot dogs per 1 lb-sized package)
Hot dog: turkey or chicken	1 hot dog (10 hot dogs per 1 lb-sized package)
Pork: sausage, spareribs	1 oz
⬛ Processed sandwich meats with 8 grams of fat or more per oz: bologna, hard salami, pastrami	1 oz
⬛ Sausage with 8 grams fat or more per oz: bratwurst, chorizo, Italian, knockwurst, Polish, smoked, summer	1 oz

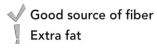 **Good source of fiber**
! **Extra fat**

⬛ **High in sodium** (based on the sodium content of a typical 3-oz serving of meat, unless 1 oz or 2 oz is the normal serving size)

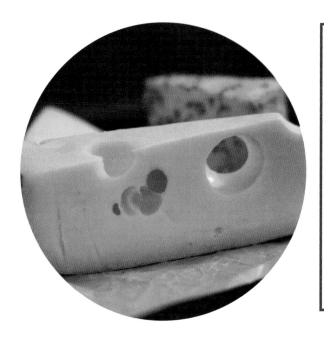

Note

- Beans, peas, and lentils are also found on the **Starch** list, page 14.
- Nut butters in smaller amounts are found in the **Fats** list, page 39.
- Canned beans, lentils, and peas can be high in sodium unless they're labeled *no-salt-added* or *low-sodium*. Draining and rinsing canned beans, peas, and lentils reduces sodium content by at least 40%.

Plant-Based Protein

Because carbohydrate content varies among plant-based protein foods, read food labels.

Food	Serving Size	Choices per Serving
"Bacon" strips, soy-based	2 strips (½ oz)	1 lean protein
✓ Baked beans, canned	⅓ cup	1 starch + 1 lean protein
✓ Beans (black, garbanzo, kidney, lima, navy, pinto, white), cooked or canned, drained and rinsed	½ cup	1 starch + 1 lean protein
"Beef" or "sausage" crumbles, meatless	1 oz	1 lean protein
"Chicken" nuggets, soy-based	2 nuggets (1½ oz)	½ carbohydrate + 1 medium-fat protein
✓ Edamame, shelled	½ cup	½ carbohydrate + 1 lean protein
Falafel (spiced chickpea and wheat patties)	3 patties (about 2 inches across)	1 carbohydrate + 1 high-fat protein
Hot dog, meatless, soy-based	1 hot dog (1½ oz)	1 lean protein
✓ Hummus	⅓ cup	1 carbohydrate + 1 medium-fat protein
✓ Lentils, any color, cooked or canned, drained and rinsed	½ cup	1 starch + 1 lean protein
Meatless burger, soy-based	3 oz	½ carbohydrate + 2 lean proteins
✓ Meatless burger, vegetable- and starch-based	1 patty (about 2½ oz)	½ carbohydrate + 1 lean protein
Meatless deli slices	1 oz	1 lean protein
Mycoprotein ("chicken" tenders or crumbles), meatless	2 oz	½ carbohydrate + 1 lean protein
Nut spreads: almond butter, cashew butter, peanut butter, soy nut butter	1 Tbsp	1 high-fat protein
✓ Peas (black-eyed and split peas), cooked or canned, drained and rinsed	½ cup	1 starch + 1 lean protein
⒮ ✓ Refried beans, canned	½ cup	1 starch + 1 lean protein
"Sausage" breakfast-type patties, meatless	1 (1½ oz)	1 medium-fat protein
Soy nuts, unsalted	¾ oz	½ carbohydrate + 1 medium-fat protein
Tempeh, plain, unflavored	¼ cup (1½ oz)	1 medium-fat protein
Tofu	½ cup (4 oz)	1 medium-fat protein
Tofu, light	½ cup (4 oz)	1 lean protein

Fats

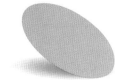

The fats on this list are divided into three groups, based on the main type of fat they contain:

- **Unsaturated fats** primarily come from vegetable sources and are considered healthy fats.
  - **Monounsaturated fats**
  - **Polyunsaturated fats** (including omega-3 fats)
- **Saturated fats** primarily come from animal sources and are considered unhealthy fats.

Trans fat, a product of food processing, is an unhealthy fat and should be avoided (see sidebar on page 38).

Nutrition Tips

- A choice on the **Fats** list contains 5 grams of fat and 45 calories. In general, **1 fat choice** equals:
  - 1 teaspoon of oil or solid fat
  - 1 tablespoon of salad dressing
- All fats are high in calories. Limit serving sizes for good nutrition and health.
- Limit the amount of fried foods you eat.
- Choose unsaturated fats instead of saturated and *trans* fats whenever possible.
- Nuts and seeds are good sources of unsaturated fats and have small amounts of fiber and protein. Eat them in moderation to control calories.
- Good sources of omega-3 fatty acids include:
  - Fish such as albacore tuna, halibut, herring, mackerel, salmon, sardines, and trout
  - Flaxseeds and English walnuts
  - Oils such as canola, soybean, flaxseed, and walnut

Selection Tips

- Check the Nutrition Facts panel on food labels for serving sizes. One fat choice is based on a serving size that has 5 grams of total fat. Remember: The label serving size may be different than the serving size used in this food list.
- The food label lists total fat grams, saturated fat grams, and *trans* fat grams per serving. When most of the total fat comes from saturated fat, the food is listed on the Saturated Fats list.

Fats

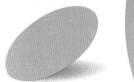

- When selecting fats, consider replacing saturated fats with monounsaturated fats and polyunsaturated fats that are good sources of omega-3 fats. Talk with your RDN about the best choices for you.
- Choose liquid oils instead of solid fats, such as butter, lard, shortening, or margarine, for cooking or baking.
- Read ingredient lists. Replace fats or spreads that include partially hydrogenated oils (*trans* fats) in the ingredient list with products containing oils that do NOT include the words "partially hydrogenated" or "hydrogenated."
- When selecting margarine, choose a type that either lists liquid vegetable oil (*trans* fat–free) as the first ingredient or lists water as the first ingredient and liquid vegetable oil as the second ingredient.
- Soft or tub margarines have less saturated fat than stick margarines and are a healthier choice. Select *trans* fat–free soft margarines.

Trans Fat

Avoid *trans* fats. Most *trans* fats found in foods are made in a process that changes vegetable oils into semi-solid fats. Partially hydrogenated and hydrogenated fats are types of processed *trans* fats and should be avoided. *Trans* fats can often be found in the following types of foods:

- Solid vegetable shortening, stick margarines, and some tub margarines
- Crackers, candies, cookies, snack foods, fried foods, baked goods, coffee creamers, and other food items made with partially hydrogenated vegetable oils

Keep in mind that some foods claiming to be *trans* fat–free may still contain *trans* fat. Foods only need to have less than ½ gram of *trans* fat per serving to be labeled *trans* fat–free.

Unsaturated Fats—Monounsaturated Fats

Food	Serving Size
Almond milk (unsweetened)	1 cup
Avocado, medium	2 Tbsp (1 oz)
Nut butters (*trans* fat–free): almond butter, cashew butter, peanut butter (smooth or crunchy)	1½ tsp
Nuts	
almonds	6 nuts
Brazil	2 nuts
cashews	6 nuts
filberts (hazelnuts)	5 nuts
macadamia	3 nuts
mixed (50% peanuts)	6 nuts
peanuts	10 nuts
pecans	4 halves
pistachios	16 nuts
Oil: canola, olive, peanut	1 tsp
Olives	
black (ripe)	8
green, stuffed	10 large
Spread, plant stanol ester–type	
light	1 Tbsp
regular	2 tsp

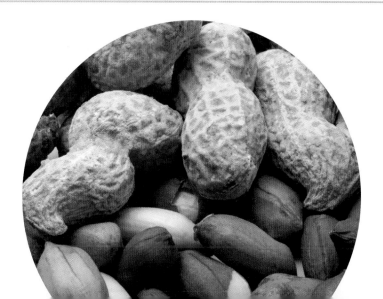

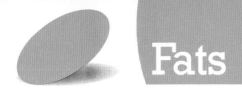

Fats

Unsaturated Fats—Polyunsaturated Fats

Food	Serving Size
Margarine	
lower-fat spread (30 to 50% vegetable oil, *trans* fat–free)	1 Tbsp
stick, tub (*trans* fat–free), or squeeze (*trans* fat–free)	1 tsp
Mayonnaise	
reduced-fat	1 Tbsp
regular	1 tsp
Mayonnaise-style salad dressing	
reduced-fat	1 Tbsp
regular	2 tsp
Nuts	
pignolia (pine nuts)	1 Tbsp
walnuts, English	4 halves
Oil: corn, cottonseed, flaxseed, grapeseed, safflower, soybean, sunflower	1 tsp
Salad dressing	
reduced-fat (Note: May contain carbohydrate.)	2 Tbsp
regular	1 Tbsp
Seeds	
flaxseed, ground	1½ Tbsp
pumpkin, sesame, sunflower	1 Tbsp
Tahini or sesame paste	2 tsp

Portion Tip

Your thumb is about the same size and volume as 1 tablespoon of salad dressing, mayonnaise, margarine, or oil. It is also about the same size as 1 ounce of cheese. A thumb tip is about the size of 1 teaspoon of margarine, mayonnaise, or other fats and oils.

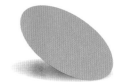

Saturated Fats

Food	Serving Size
Bacon, cooked, regular or turkey	1 slice
Butter	
reduced-fat	1 Tbsp
stick	1 tsp
whipped	2 tsp
Butter blends made with oil	
reduced-fat or light	1 Tbsp
regular	1½ tsp
Chitterlings, boiled	2 Tbsp (½ oz)
Coconut, sweetened, shredded	2 Tbsp
Coconut milk, canned, thick	
light	⅓ cup
regular	1½ Tbsp
Coconut milk beverage (thin), unsweetened	1 cup
Cream	
half-and-half	2 Tbsp
heavy	1 Tbsp
light	1½ Tbsp
whipped	2 Tbsp
Cream cheese	
reduced-fat	1½ Tbsp (¾ oz)
regular	1 Tbsp (½ oz)
Lard	1 tsp
Oil: coconut, palm, palm kernel	1 tsp
Salt pork	¼ oz
Shortening, solid	1 tsp
Sour cream	
reduced-fat or light	3 Tbsp
regular	2 Tbsp

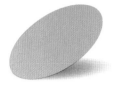

Fats

Similar Foods in Other Lists

- Bacon and nut butters, when used in smaller amounts, are counted as fat choices. When used in larger amounts, they are counted as high-fat protein choices (see the **Protein** list, pages 35).

- Fat-free salad dressings are on the **Sweets, Desserts, and Other Carbohydrates** list, page 28.

- Look for whipped topping and fat-free products, such as margarines, salad dressings, mayonnaise, sour cream, and cream cheese, on the **Free Foods** list, page 44.

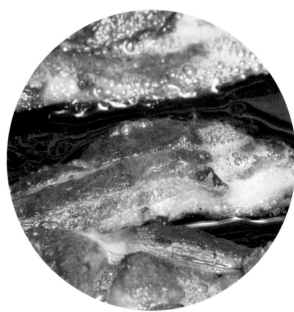

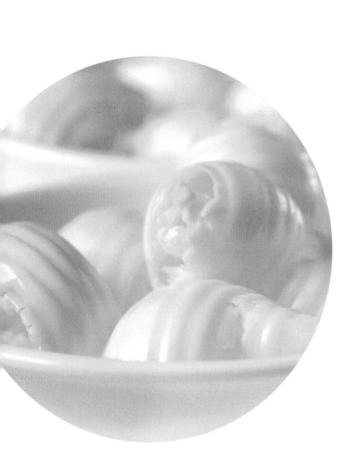

Free Foods

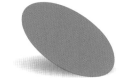

A "free" food is any food or drink choice that has less than 20 calories and 5 grams or less of carbohydrate per serving.

Nutrition Tip

- Some free foods contain sodium (salt). Examples of high-sodium seasonings or condiments include soy sauce, flavored salts (such as garlic salt and celery salt), and lemon pepper. Use these seasonings less often and in small amounts.

Selection Tips

- If a "free" food is listed with a serving size, that means the calories and/or carbohydrate are near the limits defined for "free." Limit yourself to 3 servings or fewer of that food per day, and spread the servings throughout the day. If you eat all 3 servings at once, the carbohydrate in the food may raise your blood glucose level like 1 carbohydrate choice would.
- Food and drink choices listed here without a serving size can be used whenever you like.

Low-Carbohydrate Foods

Food	Serving Size
Candy, hard (regular or sugar-free)	1 piece
Fruits	
Cranberries or rhubarb, sweetened with sugar substitute	½ cup
Gelatin dessert, sugar-free, any flavor	
Gum, sugar-free	
Jam or jelly, light or no-sugar-added	2 tsp
Salad greens (such as arugula, chicory, endive, escarole, leaf or iceberg lettuce, purslane, romaine, radicchio, spinach, watercress)	
Sugar substitutes (artificial sweeteners)	
Syrup, sugar-free	2 Tbsp
Vegetables: any **raw** nonstarchy vegetables (such as broccoli, cabbage, carrots, cucumber, tomato)	½ cup
Vegetables: any **cooked** nonstarchy vegetables (such as carrots, cauliflower, green beans)	¼ cup

Free Foods

Reduced-Fat or Fat-Free Foods

Food	Serving Size
Cream cheese, fat-free	1 Tbsp (½ oz)
Coffee creamers, nondairy	
liquid, flavored	1½ tsp
liquid, sugar-free, flavored	4 tsp
powdered, flavored	1 tsp
powdered, sugar-free, flavored	2 tsp
Margarine spread	
fat-free	1 Tbsp
reduced-fat	1 tsp
Mayonnaise	
fat-free	1 Tbsp
reduced-fat	1 tsp
Mayonnaise-style salad dressing	
fat-free	1 Tbsp
reduced-fat	2 tsp
Salad dressing	
fat-free	1 Tbsp
fat-free, Italian	2 Tbsp
Sour cream, fat-free or reduced-fat	1 Tbsp
Whipped topping	
light or fat-free	2 Tbsp
regular	1 Tbsp

Artificial Sweeteners

Sugar substitutes, alternatives, or replacements that are approved by the Food and Drug Administration (FDA) are safe to use. Each sweetener is tested for safety before it can be marketed and sold. Common types include:

- Aspartame, neotame (blue packet)
- Monk fruit (orange packet)
- Saccharin (pink packet)
- Stevia (green packet) (Note: The whole leaf or crude form of stevia is not FDA-approved.)
- Sucralose (yellow packet)

Note: Blended sweeteners (mixtures of a sweetener and sugar [sucrose]) are found in the **Sweets** list on page 28.

Condiments

Food	Serving Size
Barbecue sauce	2 tsp
Catsup (ketchup)	1 Tbsp
Chili sauce, sweet, tomato-type	2 tsp
Horseradish	
Hot pepper sauce	
Lemon juice	
Miso	1½ tsp
Mustard	
honey	1 Tbsp
brown, Dijon, horseradish-flavored, wasabi-flavored, or yellow	
Parmesan cheese, grated	1 Tbsp
Pickle relish (dill or sweet)	1 Tbsp
Pickles	
dill	1½ medium pickles
sweet, bread and butter	2 slices
sweet, gherkin	¾ oz
Pimento	
Salsa	¼ cup
Soy sauce, light or regular	1 Tbsp
Sweet-and-sour sauce	2 tsp
Taco sauce	1 Tbsp
Vinegar	
Worcestershire sauce	
Yogurt, any type	2 Tbsp

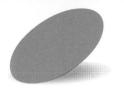

Free Foods

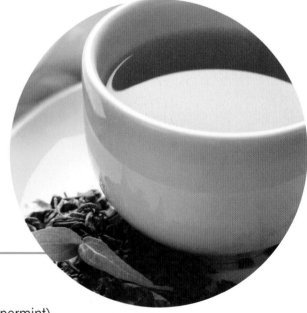

Free Snack Suggestions

When you are hungry between meals, try to choose whole foods as snacks instead of highly processed options. The foods listed below are examples of healthy free-food snacks:

- ½ choice from the **Nonstarchy Vegetables** list on page 24; for example, ½ cup raw broccoli, carrots, celery, cucumber, or tomato
- ⅓ choice from the **Fruits** list on pages 16–17; for example, ¼ cup blueberries or blackberries, ⅓ cup melon, 6 grapes, or 2 tsp dried fruits
- ¼ choice from the **Starch** list on pages 9–13; for example, 2 animal crackers, 1½ saltine-type crackers, ¾ cup no-fat-added popcorn, or ½ regular-sized rice or popcorn cake
- ½ choice from the nuts and seeds portion of the **Fats** list on pages 39–40; for example, 8 pistachios, 3 almonds, 4 black olives, or 1½ tsp sunflower seeds
- ½ choice from the **Lean Protein** list on page 33; for example, ½ oz slice of fat-free cheese or ½ oz of lean cooked meat

Drinks/Mixes

- Bouillon, broth, consommé
- Bouillon or broth, low-sodium
- Carbonated or mineral water
- Club soda
- Cocoa powder, unsweetened (1 Tbsp)
- Coffee, unsweetened or with sugar substitute
- Diet soft drinks, sugar-free
- Drink mixes (powder or liquid drops), sugar-free
- Tea, unsweetened or with sugar substitute
- Tonic water, sugar-free
- Water
- Water, flavored, sugar-free

Seasonings

- Flavoring extracts (for example, vanilla, almond, or peppermint)
- Garlic, fresh or powder
- Herbs, fresh or dried
- Kelp
- Nonstick cooking spray
- Spices
- Wine, used in cooking

Combination Foods

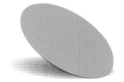

Many of the foods you eat, such as casseroles and frozen entrees, are mixed together in various combinations. These "combination" foods do not fit into any one choice list. This list of some typical "combination" food choices will help you fit these foods into your Eating Plan. Ask your RDN about the nutrient information for other combination foods you would like to eat, including your own recipes. One carbohydrate choice in this list has 15 grams of carbohydrate and about 70 calories.

Entrees

	Food	Serving Size	Choices per Serving
🧂	Casserole-type entrees (tuna noodle, lasagna, spaghetti with meatballs, chili with beans, macaroni and cheese)	1 cup (8 oz)	2 carbohydrates + 2 medium-fat proteins
🧂	Stews (beef/other meats and vegetables)	1 cup (8 oz)	1 carbohydrate + 1 medium-fat protein + 0 to 3 fats

Frozen Meals/Entrees

	Food	Serving Size	Choices per Serving
🧂✓	Burrito (beef and bean)	1 burrito (5 oz)	3 carbohydrates + 1 lean protein + 2 fats
	Dinner-type healthy meal (includes dessert and is usually less than 400 calories)	about 9–12 oz	2 to 3 carbohydrates + 1 to 2 lean proteins + 1 fat
	"Healthy"-type entree (usually less than 300 calories)	about 7–10 oz	2 carbohydrates + 2 lean proteins
	Pizza		
🧂	cheese/vegetarian, thin crust	¼ of a 12-inch pizza (4½–5 oz)	2 carbohydrates + 2 medium-fat proteins
🧂	meat topping, thin crust	¼ of a 12-inch pizza (5 oz)	2 carbohydrates + 2 medium-fat proteins + 1½ fats
🧂	cheese/vegetarian or meat topping, rising crust	⅙ of 12-inch pizza (4 oz)	2½ carbohydrates + 2 medium-fat proteins
🧂	Pocket sandwich	1 sandwich (4½ oz)	3 carbohydrates + 1 lean protein + 1 to 2 fats
🧂	Pot pie	1 pot pie (7 oz)	3 carbohydrates + 1 medium-fat protein + 3 fats

✓ **Good source of fiber**   ❗ **Extra fat**   🧂 **High in sodium**   *Combination Foods*   **47**

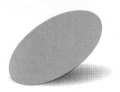

Combination Foods

Salads (Deli-Style)

Food	Serving Size	Choices per Serving
Coleslaw	½ cup	1 carbohydrate + 1½ fats
Macaroni/pasta salad	½ cup	2 carbohydrates + 3 fats
Potato salad	½ cup	1½ to 2 carbohydrates + 1 to 2 fats
Tuna salad or chicken salad	½ cup (3½ oz)	½ carbohydrate + 2 lean proteins + 1 fat

Soups

Food	Serving Size	Choices per Serving
Bean, lentil, or split pea soup	1 cup (8 oz)	1½ carbohydrates + 1 lean protein
Chowder (made with milk)	1 cup (8 oz)	1 carbohydrate + 1 lean protein + 1½ fats
Cream soup (made with water)	1 cup (8 oz)	1 carbohydrate + 1 fat
Miso soup	1 cup (8 oz)	½ carbohydrate + 1 lean protein
Ramen noodle soup	1 cup (8 oz)	2 carbohydrates + 2 fats
Rice soup/porridge (congee)	1 cup (8 oz)	1 carbohydrate
Tomato soup (made with water), borscht	1 cup (8 oz)	1 carbohydrate
Vegetable beef, chicken noodle, or other broth-type soup (including "healthy"-type soups, such as those lower in sodium and/or fat)	1 cup (8 oz)	1 carbohydrate + 1 lean protein

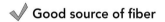 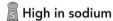

✓ Good source of fiber   ! Extra fat   Ⓢ High in sodium

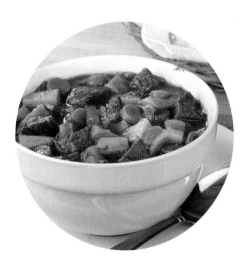 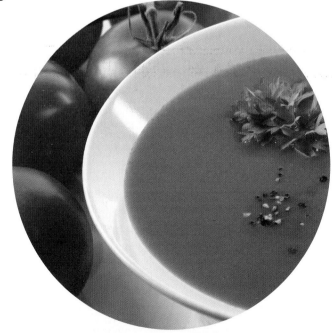

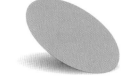

Other Combination Foods

The nutrient content of your home recipes may be different from the carbohydrate, protein, and fat choices that are listed here for similar combination foods. To figure out the nutrient content of a recipe, follow these steps:

- Find the carbohydrate grams, protein grams, fat grams, and calorie information for each ingredient. (For packaged foods, this information is on the Nutrition Facts panel on the label.)
- Figure out the total amount of calories and total amount of each of the nutrients for the recipe.
- Divide the totals for calories and each nutrient by the number of servings the recipe yields.
- Compare these numbers with the definitions of carbohydrate, protein, and fat choices in this booklet. For example, if 1 serving of the recipe has 30 grams of carbohydrate and 10 grams of fat, count that serving as 2 carbohydrate choices and 2 fat choices.

For more information on finding nutrients for ingredients, read the Reading Food Labels section on page 56 or use the American Diabetes Association's My Food Advisor™ website: http://tracker.diabetes.org/.

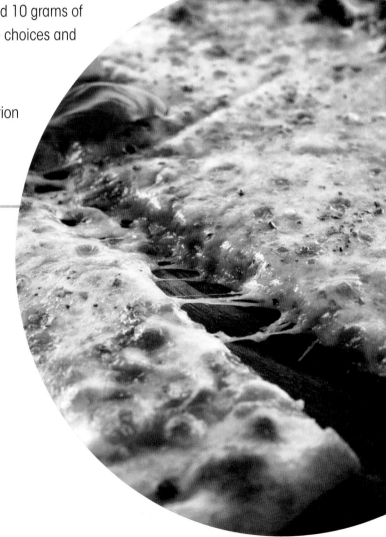

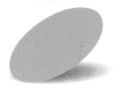

Fast Foods

The choices in the **Fast Foods** list are not specific fast food meals or items, but are estimates based on popular foods. You can get specific nutrition information for almost every fast food or restaurant chain. Ask the restaurant or check its website for nutrition information about your favorite fast foods. One carbohydrate choice has 15 grams of carbohydrate and about 70 calories.

Eating Out and Eating Healthy

- Plan ahead. Make a list of restaurants near you that offer healthy choices and pick up carryout menus or check the menus on their websites.
- Ask questions before you place your order: How is the item prepared? Can you substitute items?
- Ask your server not to bring bread or chips to the table before your meal.
- Ask for more vegetables whenever possible.
- Avoid items that are "jumbo," "giant," "deluxe," or "super-sized."
- Split an entree or dessert with someone.
- Put half of your order in a take-home box before you start to eat.
- Watch out for foods that contain extra calories, such as croutons, bacon, or cheese.
- Ask for salad dressings, sour cream, and butter on the side so you can control the amount used.
- Don't forget to count calories and carbohydrates in beverages.
- Walk (or ride your bike) to and from the restaurant to burn extra calories.

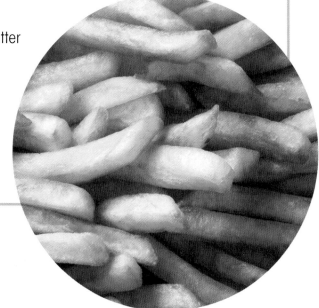

Main Dishes/Entrees

	Food	Serving Size	Choices per Serving
	Chicken		
🧂	breast, breaded and fried*	1 (about 7 oz)	1 carbohydrate + 6 medium-fat proteins
	breast, meat only**	1	4 lean proteins
	drumstick, breaded and fried*	1 (about 2½ oz)	½ carbohydrate + 2 medium-fat proteins
	drumstick, meat only**	1	1 lean protein + ½ fat
🧂	nuggets or tenders	6 (about 3½ oz)	1 carbohydrate + 2 medium-fat proteins + 1 fat
🧂	thigh, breaded and fried*	1 (about 5 oz)	1 carbohydrate + 3 medium-fat proteins + 2 fats
	thigh, meat only**	1	2 lean proteins + ½ fat
	wing, breaded and fried*	1 wing (about 2 oz)	½ carbohydrate + 2 medium-fat proteins
	wing, meat only**	1 wing	1 lean protein
🧂✓	Main dish salad (grilled chicken-type, no dressing or croutons)	1 salad (about 11½ oz)	1 carbohydrate + 4 lean proteins
	Pizza		
🧂	cheese, pepperoni, or sausage, regular or thick crust	⅛ of a 14-inch pizza (about 4 oz)	2½ carbohydrates + 1 high-fat protein + 1 fat
🧂	cheese, pepperoni, or sausage, thin crust	⅛ of a 14-inch pizza (about 2¾ oz)	1½ carbohydrates + 1 high-fat protein + 1 fats
🧂	cheese, meat, and vegetable, regular crust	⅛ of a 14-inch pizza (about 5 oz)	2½ carbohydrates + 2 high-fat proteins

*Definition and weight refer to food **with** bone, skin, and breading.
Definition refers to above food **without bone, skin, and breading.

✓ Good source of fiber   ❗ Extra fat   🧂 High in sodium

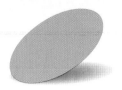

Fast Foods

Asian

	Food	Serving Size	Choices per Serving
S	Beef/chicken/shrimp with vegetables in sauce	1 cup (about 6 oz)	1 carbohydrate + 2 lean proteins + 1 fat
	Egg roll, meat	1 egg roll (about 3 oz)	1½ carbohydrates + 1 lean protein + 1½ fats
	Fried rice, meatless	1 cup	2½ carbohydrates + 2 fats
	Fortune cookie	1 cookie	½ carbohydrate
S	Hot-and-sour soup	1 cup	½ carbohydrate + ½ fat
S	Meat with sweet sauce	1 cup (about 6 oz)	3½ carbohydrates + 3 medium-fat proteins + 3 fats
S	Noodles and vegetables in sauce (chow mein, lo mein)	1 cup	2 carbohydrates + 2 fats

Mexican

	Food	Serving Size	Choices per Serving
S ✓	Burrito with beans and cheese	1 small burrito (about 6 oz)	3½ carbohydrates + 1 medium-fat protein + 1 fat
S	Nachos with cheese	1 small order (about 8 nachos)	2½ carbohydrates + 1 high-fat protein + 2 fats
S	Quesadilla, cheese only	1 small order (about 5 oz)	2½ carbohydrates + 3 high-fat proteins
	Taco, crisp, with meat and cheese	1 small taco (about 3 oz)	1 carbohydrate + 1 medium-fat protein + ½ fat
S ✓	Taco salad with chicken and tortilla bowl	1 salad (1 lb, including tortilla bowl)	3½ carbohydrates + 4 medium-fat proteins + 3 fats
S	Tostada with beans and cheese	1 small tostada (about 5 oz)	2 carbohydrates + 1 high-fat protein

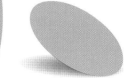

Sandwiches

Food	Serving Size	Choices per Serving
Breakfast Sandwiches		
Breakfast burrito with sausage, egg, cheese	1 burrito (about 4 oz)	1½ carbohydrates + 2 high-fat proteins
Egg, cheese, meat on an English muffin	1 sandwich	2 carbohydrates + 3 medium-fat proteins + ½ fat
Egg, cheese, meat on a biscuit	1 sandwich	2 carbohydrates + 3 medium-fat proteins + 2 fats
Sausage biscuit sandwich	1 sandwich	2 carbohydrates + 1 high-fat protein + 4 fats
Chicken Sandwiches		
grilled with bun, lettuce, tomatoes, spread	1 sandwich (about 7½ oz)	3 carbohydrates + 4 lean proteins
crispy, with bun, lettuce, tomatoes, spread	1 sandwich (about 6 oz)	3 carbohydrates + 2 lean proteins + 3½ fats
Fish sandwich with tartar sauce and cheese	1 sandwich (5 oz)	2½ carbohydrates + 2 medium-fat proteins + 1½ fats
Hamburger		
regular with bun and condiments (catsup, mustard, onion, pickle)	1 burger (about 3½ oz)	2 carbohydrates + 1 medium-fat protein + 1 fat
4 oz meat with cheese, bun, and condiments (catsup, mustard, onion, pickle)	1 burger (about 8½ oz)	3 carbohydrates + 4 medium-fat protein + 2½ fats
Hot dog with bun, plain	1 hot dog (about 3½ oz)	1½ carbohydrates + 1 high-fat protein + 2 fats
Submarine sandwich (no cheese or sauce)		
less than 6 grams fat	1 6-inch sub	3 carbohydrates + 2 lean proteins
regular	1 6-inch sub	3 carbohydrates + 2 lean proteins + 1 fat
Wrap, grilled chicken, vegetables, cheese, and spread	1 small wrap (about 4 to 5 oz)	2 carbohydrates + 2 lean proteins + 1½ fats

✓ Good source of fiber   ▮ Extra fat   🧂 High in sodium

Fast Foods

Sides/Appetizers

	Food	Serving Size	Choices per Serving
🧂!	French fries	1 small order (about 3½ oz)	2½ carbohydrates + 2 fats
		1 medium order (about 5 oz)	3½ carbohydrates + 3 fats
		1 large order (about 6 oz)	4½ carbohydrates + 4 fats
🧂	Hashbrowns	1 cup/medium order (about 5 oz)	3 carbohydrates + 6 fats
🧂	Onion rings	1 serving (8 to 9 rings, about 4 oz)	3½ carbohydrates + 4 fats
	Salad, side (no dressing, croutons or cheese)	1 small salad	1 nonstarchy vegetable

Beverages and Desserts

Food	Serving Size	Choices per Serving
Coffee, latte (fat-free milk)	1 small order (about 12 oz)	1 fat-free milk
Coffee, mocha (fat-free milk, no whipped cream)	1 small order (about 12 oz)	1 fat-free milk + 1 carbohydrate
Milkshake, any flavor	1 small shake (about 12 oz)	5½ carbohydrates + 3 fats
	1 medium shake (about 16 oz)	7 carbohydrates + 4 fats
	1 large shake (about 22 oz)	10 carbohydrates + 5 fats
Soft-serve ice cream cone	1 small	2 carbohydrates + ½ fat

Note: See the **Starch** list for plain rice; see the **Starch** list and **Sweets, Desserts, and Other Carbohydrates** list for foods such as bagels and muffins; see the **Starch** list or **Protein** list for refried and other beans; see the **Sweets, Desserts, and Other Carbohydrates** list for frozen desserts such as ice cream or frozen yogurt.

Alcohol

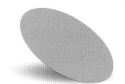

Nutrition Tips

- In general, 1 alcohol equivalent (½ oz absolute alcohol, also known as ethanol or ethyl alcohol) has about 100 calories.

Selection Tips

- Women who choose to drink alcohol should limit alcohol to 1 serving or less per day. Men who choose to drink alcohol should limit alcohol to 2 servings or less per day.
- To reduce your risk of low blood glucose (hypoglycemia), especially if you take insulin or a diabetes pill that increases insulin, never drink alcohol on an empty stomach. Always eat a carbohydrate food when you are having an alcoholic beverage.
- While alcohol does not directly affect blood glucose levels, be aware of the carbohydrate in alcoholic beverages, such as mixed drinks, beer, and wine. The carbohydrate may raise your blood glucose levels.
- Check with your RDN if you would like to fit alcohol into your Eating Plan.

One alcohol equivalent or choice (½ oz absolute alcohol) has about 100 calories.
One carbohydrate choice has 15 grams of carbohydrate and about 70 calories.

Alcoholic Beverage	Serving Size	Choices per Serving
Beer		
light (less than 4.5% abv)	12 fl oz	1 alcohol equivalent + ½ carbohydrate
regular (about 5% abv)	12 fl oz	1 alcohol equivalent + 1 carbohydrate
dark (more than 5.7% abv)	12 fl oz	1 alcohol equivalent + 1 to 1½ carbohydrates
Distilled spirits (80 or 86 proof): vodka, rum, gin, whiskey, tequila	1½ fl oz	1 alcohol equivalent
Liqueur, coffee (53 proof)	1 fl oz	½ alcohol equivalent + 1 carbohydrate
Sake	1 fl oz	½ alcohol equivalent
Wine		
champagne/sparkling	5 fl oz	1 alcohol equivalent
dessert (sherry)	3½ fl oz	1 alcohol equivalent + 1 carbohydrate
dry, red or white (10% abv)	5 fl oz	1 alcohol equivalent

Note: The abbreviation "% abv" refers to the percentage of alcohol by volume.

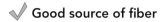 Good source of fiber   Extra fat   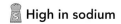 High in sodium

Reading Food Labels

Checking the Nutrition Facts panel and ingredients list on a food label can help you with your food choices. For more help using the information on food labels, ask your RDN.

Check the Serving Size. All the other information in the Nutrition Facts panel will be for 1 serving of this size. Note: For some foods, the serving on the label is not the same size that is used in this booklet. When counting servings in your Eating Plan, use the serving sizes from this booklet.

Look at the Calories per serving. A serving with less than 20 calories and less than 5 grams of carbohydrate may be counted as a "free food." If the food has more than 20 calories per serving, count the carbohydrate, protein, and fat choices to know how the food fits in your Eating Plan.

Check the amount of sodium to see how the food fits within your daily limits for sodium.

Look for foods that are rich in these nutrients to get the most nutrition for your calories.

Nutrition Facts

Serving Size 1 cup (240g)
Servings Per Container 2

Amount Per Serving

Calories 230   **Calories from Fat** 70

	% Daily Value*
Total Fat 8g	**12%**
Saturated Fat 3.5g	18%
Trans Fat 0.5g	
Cholesterol 30mg	**10%**
Sodium 870mg	**36%**
Total Carbohydrate 25g	**8%**
Dietary Fiber 8g	**32%**
Sugars 11g	
Protein 15g	

Vitamin A 10%	•	Vitamin C 2%
Calcium 4%	•	Iron 10%

*Percent Daily Values are based on a 2,000 calorie diet. Your Daily Values may be higher or lower depending on your calorie needs.

	Calories:	2,000	2,500
Total Fat	Less than	65g	80g
Sat Fat	Less than	20g	25g
Cholesterol	Less than	300mg	300mg
Sodium	Less than	2,400mg	2,400mg
Total Carbohydrate		300g	375g
Dietary Fiber		25g	30g

Ingredients: water, tomato puree (water, tomato paste), seasoned beef crumbles (beef, salt, spice extracts), diced tomatoes in tomato juice, red kidney beans, kidney beans. Contains less than 2% of the following ingredients: concentrate (caramel color added), jalapeno peppers, salt, dehydrated onions, **sugar**, dehydrated garlic, paprika, red pepper, soybean oil, soy lecithin, mono and diglycerides, mixed tocopherols, ascorbic acid, flavoring.

Look at the grams of Total Fat in 1 serving. Use this information to figure out how many fat choices are in 1 serving (1 fat choice has 5 grams of fat).

To help lower your risk of heart disease, **choose foods that are low in saturated fat and cholesterol and have zero *trans* fat**.

Check the grams of Total Carbohydrate in 1 serving. Total carbohydrate includes the grams of dietary fiber and sugars. To figure out how many carbohydrate choices are in 1 serving, divide the Total Carbohydrate by 15 (1 carbohydrate choice has 15 grams of carbohydrate). You may need to adjust the size of the serving to fit with the carbohydrate choices in your Eating Plan.

Look for foods rich in Dietary Fiber. A good source of fiber has about 3 grams per serving. An excellent source has at least 5 grams per serving.

Choose foods that are low in added Sugars. Every 4 grams of sugar is equal to 1 teaspoon. The sugars listed on the Nutrition Facts panel include both naturally occurring sugars (such as in fruit and dairy products) and those that are added. To determine if added sugars are in the product, **check the ingredients list** for these added-sugar words: added sugars (brown, confectioner's, powdered, turbinado, cane, date, invert), sucrose, polydextrose, fructose, maltose, dextrose, syrup (corn, maple, agave), honey, molasses, and agave nectar. If you see any of these words among the first few ingredients on the list, then the food is high in added sugars.

Nutrient Content Claims

The health claims printed on food and drink packaging are regulated by the Food and Drug Administration (FDA) and must meet certain guidelines. Here are definitions of some popular claims:

- **Reduced-fat** means the food or drink has at least 25% less fat per serving than a comparable regular food or drink.
- **Low-fat** means the food or drink has 3 grams or less of fat per serving.
- **Fat-free** means the food or drink has less than $1/2$ gram of fat per serving.
- **_Trans_ fat–free** means the food or drink has less than $1/2$ gram of _trans_ fat per serving. (Note: The Nutrition Facts panel on the label will list 0g [zero grams] _trans_ fat for any food with less than $1/2$ gram of _trans_ fat per serving. To know whether a food has any _trans_ fat, check the ingredients list. If the ingredients include hydrogenated or partially hydrogenated oil, then the food contains some _trans_ fat—regardless of the labeling claim.)
- **Light** can mean the food or drink has at least $1/3$ fewer calories per serving than a comparable regular food or drink, **or** it can mean the food or drink has at least 50% less fat per serving than a comparable regular food or drink.
- **Reduced-calorie** means the food or drink has at least 25% fewer calories per serving than a comparable regular food or drink.
- **Sugar-free** means the food or drink has less than $1/2$ gram of sugar per serving.

Tips for Sugar Alcohols

- To find out if a product contains sugar alcohols (which are often found in sugar-free baked goods and candies), check the food label carefully. Sugar alcohol is sometimes listed below sugars on the Nutrition Facts panel on the label. You can also check the ingredients list for erythritol, glycerol, hydrogenated starch hydrolysate, isomalt, lactitol, maltitol, mannitol, sorbitol, and xylitol. (These are types of sugar alcohols.)
- Foods with sugar alcohols can affect blood glucose levels. When you eat foods with sugar alcohols, check your blood glucose to note their effect on you.
- Sugar alcohols may cause bloating, gas, or diarrhea, especially in children, although not everyone experiences these problems.

Glossary

A1C: A test that measures average blood glucose level over the past 2 to 3 months, usually shown as a percentage. Also called hemoglobin A1C or glycosylated hemoglobin, the test shows the amount of glucose that sticks to red blood cells, which represents the amount of glucose in the blood. The American Diabetes Association recommends an A1C goal of <7% for nonpregnant adults with diabetes. A1C goals may need to be higher for individuals with hypoglycemia unawareness, young children, the elderly, or people with a history of significant heart disease.

Alcohol: An ingredient in a variety of drinks, including beer, wine, liqueurs, cordials, and mixed or straight drinks. Pure alcohol has about 7 calories per gram.

Blood glucose (also called **blood sugar**): The main sugar found in the blood and the body's main energy source.

Blood glucose level: The amount of glucose in a given amount of blood is measured in milligrams of glucose per deciliter of blood and is shown as mg/dL. The American Diabetes Association recommends the following blood glucose goals for nonpregnant adults with diabetes:
- Fasting: 70 to 130 mg/dL
- One to two hours after the beginning of a meal: <180 mg/dL

Calorie: A unit used to measure the heat or energy value of food. Calories come from carbohydrate, protein, fat, and alcohol.

Carbohydrate: Along with fat and protein, one of the three major nutrients. Starch, sugars, and fiber are types of carbohydrate in foods. Starch is in breads, pasta, cereals, potatoes, beans, peas, and lentils. Naturally present sugars are in fruits, milk, and vegetables. Added sugars (such as granulated sugar) are in desserts, candy, jams, and syrups. Fiber is naturally occurring in plant foods. All types of carbohydrate have 4 calories per gram and can raise blood glucose levels. The amount of carbohydrate eaten at a meal or snack and available insulin in the body determine after-meal blood glucose. Therefore, monitoring the amount of carbohydrate in meals and snacks is a key strategy for blood glucose control.

Certified diabetes educator (CDE): A certified diabetes educator (CDE) is a medical/health care professional who specializes in the management of diabetes, prediabetes, and diabetes prevention. The role of a CDE is to educate and support people affected by diabetes. CDEs have passed a certification exam, stay up-to-date on diabetes care, and can help patients manage diabetes.

Choice: In this booklet foods are grouped together in lists according to similarities in food values. A single food and its given serving size within a list contains approximately the same carbohydrate, protein, fat, and calories as any of the other foods and their given serving sizes in the same list. This means that you will get the same food value if you trade one food on the list with another food on the same list. Thus a food and its serving size become a *choice* within a particular list. An Eating Plan may contain 1, 2, or even more choices from a list for a particular meal or snack.

Cholesterol (food): Food cholesterol is found in all animal products and is high in egg yolks and organ meats. Eating foods high in cholesterol and saturated fat can raise blood (serum) cholesterol levels. Foods from plants, such as fruits, vegetables, grains, beans, peas, and lentils, do not have cholesterol. Cholesterol is found in foods on the **Milk and Milk Substitutes** list, **Protein** list, and **Fats** list.

Cholesterol (serum or blood): A fat-like substance normally found in blood. A high level of cholesterol in the blood is a major risk factor for developing heart disease.

Diabetes: A condition in which the body cannot produce insulin, doesn't produce enough insulin, or cannot use the insulin it produces well. Diabetes causes the body to be unable to use glucose for energy, which results in high blood glucose levels.

Dietary fiber: Nondigestible carbohydrate from plants. Soluble fiber, a type of dietary fiber found in oats, peas, beans, apples, citrus fruits, carrots, and barley can help lower blood glucose and cholesterol levels. The Institute of Medicine recommends that adults eat 21 grams to 38 grams of total fiber per day.

Eating Plan: A guide showing the number of food choices to have in each meal and snack. An Eating Plan helps spread carbohydrate, protein, fat, and calories throughout the day.

Fat: Along with carbohydrate and protein, one of the three major energy sources in food. Fat has 9 calories per gram, more than twice the calories provided by carbohydrate and protein. Fat is in foods like margarine, butter, oils, salad dressings, nuts, seeds, milk, cheese, meat, fish, poultry, snack foods, ice cream, and desserts. Major sources of fat are found in foods on the **Fats** list and **Protein** list. Some foods on the **Starch** list, **Milk and Milk Substitutes** list, and **Sweets, Desserts, and Other Carbohydrates** list also have fat.

Glucose (food): A simple form of carbohydrate (monosaccharide) that is sometimes called dextrose. It is a part of most sugars that are eaten.

Gram: A unit of mass and weight in the metric system. One ounce is about 30 grams.

HDL: High-density lipoprotein, a part of the total cholesterol measurement. HDL is sometimes referred to as "good" cholesterol.

The recommended HDL level for people with diabetes is more than 40 mg/dL for men and more than 50 mg/dL for women.

Insulin: A hormone made by the pancreas that helps the body use glucose for energy. It is also a laboratory-processed medicine used by people who do not make enough of their own insulin.

LDL: Low-density lipoprotein, a part of the total cholesterol measurement. LDL is sometimes referred to as "bad" cholesterol. The recommended LDL level for people with diabetes is less than 100 mg/dL (or less than 70 mg/dL in individuals with heart disease).

Minerals: Substances essential in small amounts to build and repair body tissue and control functions of the body. Calcium, iron, magnesium, phosphorus, potassium, sodium, and zinc are minerals.

Nutrient: Substance in food necessary for life. Carbohydrate, protein, fat, minerals, vitamins, and water are all nutrients.

Prediabetes: A condition in which blood glucose levels are higher than normal but are not high enough for a diagnosis of diabetes. People with prediabetes are at increased risk for developing type 2 diabetes and for heart disease and stroke. However, a healthy Eating Plan, weight loss, and physical activity can delay or prevent development of these more serious conditions. Other names for prediabetes are impaired glucose tolerance and impaired fasting glucose.

Protein: Along with carbohydrate and fat, one of the three major nutrients in food. The body uses protein for growth, maintenance, and energy. Protein provides about 4 calories per gram. Protein is found in foods from the **Milk and Milk Substitutes** list and **Protein** list. Smaller amounts of protein are found in foods from the **Nonstarchy Vegetables** list and **Starch** list.

Registered dietitian nutritionist (RDN) or registered dietitian (RD): An RDN (or RD) is a health professional who focuses on nutrition care, education, and counseling. The initials "RDN" or "RD" after a dietitian's name ensure that she or he has met the standards of the Commission on Dietetic Registration.

Self-monitoring of blood glucose (SMBG): A self-test that determines the amount of glucose in the blood. A drop of blood is obtained by sticking the fingertip or alternate test site, such as the forearm, with a small lancet (needle). Self-monitoring of blood glucose levels on a regular basis helps people manage their diabetes.

Serving (serving size): A helping (amount) of food or drink.

Sodium: A mineral needed in small amounts by the body to maintain life. Sodium is mainly found in processed foods or table salt. Cutting down the amount of sodium in the Eating Plan may help control high blood pressure.

Starch: A type of carbohydrate with many glucose units attached together in long straight or branched chains. Foods that are made up of mostly starch are found in the **Starch** list on page 7.

Sugar alcohols (also known as **polyols**): A type of carbohydrate used as a sweetener or fat replacement. Sugar alcohols have fewer calories than sugar (2 calories per gram instead of 4 calories per gram) and cause lower after-meal blood glucose responses because the body does not fully digest them. Foods that have sugar alcohols can be labeled as "sugar-free," but that doesn't mean they are carbohydrate-free or calorie-free. Sugar alcohols include erythritol, hydrogenated starch hydrolysates, isomalt, lactitol, maltitol, mannitol, sorbitol, and xylitol.

Sugars: A type of carbohydrate having one unit (monosaccharide, a molecule such as glucose or fructose) or two attached units (such as sucrose). Sugars occur naturally in foods from the **Milk and Milk Substitutes** list, the **Nonstarchy Vegetables** list, and **Fruits** list. Added sugars (for example common table sugar, also known as sucrose, and sugar alcohols such as sorbitol) are incorporated into foods during processing and preparation.

Triglycerides: A type of fat in the blood. High triglyceride levels can increase risk for heart disease.

Vitamins: Substances found in food that are needed in small amounts to help with body processes and functions. These include vitamins A, C, D, E, and K, as well as the B-complex vitamins.

Index

Cornbread, 9
Corned beef, 34
Cornish hen, 33
Corn oil, 40
Cottage cheese, 33
Cottonseed oil, 40
Couscous, 11
Crabs, 33
Crackers, 4, 7, 13, 38, 46
Cranberries, 16, 43
Cranberry juice cocktail, 26
Cranberry sauce, 28
Cream, 19, 41
Cream cheese, 41, 42, 44
Creamers, 44
Cream soup, 48
Crispbread, 13
Croutons, 23, 50
Cucumbers, 23, 24, 43, 46
Cupcakes, 27
Curry sauce, 28
Custard pie, 27

D
Daikon, 24
Danish, 29
Dasheen, 12
Dates, 16
Dijon mustard, 45
Distilled spirits, 55
Doughnuts, 29
Dove, 34
Dried fruits, 15, 16, 46
Drink mixes, 46
Duck, 33, 34

E
Edamame, 36
Eggnog, 21
Eggplant, 23, 24
Egg rolls, 52
Eggs, 30, 34, 53
Egg substitutes, 33
Egg whites, 33
Endive, 24, 43
English muffins, 9, 53
English walnuts, 37, 40
Evaporated milk, 20

F
Falafel, 36
Fennel, 24

Feta cheese, 34
Figs, 16
Filberts (hazelnuts), 39
Fish, 30, 31, 32, 33, 34, 37, 53
Fish, fried, 30, 34
Fish sandwich, 53
Flan, 27
Flavoring extracts, 46
Flaxseed oil, 37, 40
Flaxseeds, 37, 40
Flounder, 33
Fortune cookies, 52
French-fried potato, 12
French fries, 54
Fried rice, 52
Frozen pops, 29
Fruit cobbler, 27
Fruit cocktail, 16
Fruit drink, 26
Fruit juice, 15, 18
Fruit juice bars, frozen, 29
Fruit snacks, chewy, 28
Fruit spreads, 28

G
Game, 33
Garbanzo beans, 14, 36
Garlic, 46
Garlic salt, 43
Gelatin, 27, 43
Gin, 55
Gingersnaps, 27
Goat cheese, 35
Goat's milk, 20
Goose, 33, 34
Gourds (bitter, bottle, luffa, bitter
    melon), 24
Graham crackers, 13
Granola, 10
Granola or snack bars, 13
Grapefruit, 16
Grapefruit juice, 18
Grape juice, 18
Grapes, 16, 46
Grape seed oil, 40
Gravy, canned or bottled, 28
Greek yogurt, 19, 20, 29
Green beans, 3, 24, 43
Green onions, 24
Greens (collard, dandelion,
    mustard, purslane, turnip), 24
Grits, 10

Ground beef, 32, 33, 34
Ground turkey, 33
Guava, 16
Gum, 43

H
Haddock, 33
Halibut, 30, 33, 37
Ham, 33
Hamburger, 53
Hamburger bun, 9
Hashbrowns, 54
Hazelnuts, 39
Heart, 33
Hearts of palm, 24
Herbs, 46
Herring, 30, 33, 37
Hoisin sauce, 28
Hominy, 12
Honey, 28
Honeydew melon, 17
Honey mustard, 45
Horseradish, 45
Hot-and-sour soup, 52
Hot chocolate, 26
Hot dog, 31, 33, 35, 53
Hot dog, soy-based, 36
Hot dog bun, 9
Hot pepper sauce, 45
Hummus, 36

I
Ice cream, 19, 29, 54
Imitation shellfish, 33
Instant soup, 48
Italian beans, 24
Italian sausage, 35

J
Jam or jelly, 28, 43
Jicama, 24

K
Kale, 22, 24
Kasha, 11
Kefir, 20
Kelp, 46
Kidney, 33
Kidney beans, 14, 36
Kiwi, 17
Knockwurst, 35
Kohlrabi, 22, 24